CRACKING THE CANCER CODE

CRACKING THE CANCER CODE

The SECRET to TRANSFORMING your HEALTH from Inside Out

DR. MATTHEW J. LOOP

iUniverse, Inc.
New York Lincoln Shanghai

Cracking the Cancer Code
The SECRET to TRANSFORMING your HEALTH from Inside Out

Copyright © 2006 by Matthew J. Loop

iUniverse books may be ordered through booksellers or by contacting:

iUniverse
2021 Pine Lake Road, Suite 100
Lincoln, NE 68512
www.iuniverse.com
1-800-Authors (1-800-288-4677)

The information, ideas and suggestions in this book are not intended as a substitute for professional medical advice. Before following any suggestions contained in this book, you should first consult your personal physician.

Neither the author nor the publisher shall be liable or responsible for any loss or damage allegedly arising as a consequence of your use or application of any information or suggestions in this book.

ISBN-13: 978-0-595-40169-7 (pbk)
ISBN-13: 978-0-595-67783-2 (cloth)
ISBN-13: 978-0-595-84547-7 (ebk)
ISBN-10: 0-595-40169-4 (pbk)
ISBN-10: 0-595-67783-5 (cloth)
ISBN-10: 0-595-84547-9 (ebk)

Printed in the United States of America

For my dearest Elizabeth, family and friends

Health begins with knowledge. Knowledge provides the power to take-back your health from those profiteers of disease. My intention for this book is to create a positive impact by assisting in the liberation of your mind in order to overcome adversity.

CONTENTS

Introduction xiii

Part I

CHAPTER 1   Cancer at a Glance. 3

CHAPTER 2   The Business of Healthcare 7

CHAPTER 3   A New Perspective on Health & Disease 12

CHAPTER 4   The Standard American Diet (SAD) 18

CHAPTER 5   Public Health Hazards Exposed. 23

CHAPTER 6   Modern Society Pays a Heavy Price. 28

CHAPTER 7   The Essentials of Health and Healing 30

Part II

CHAPTER 8   Everything in the Universe is Energy. 47

CHAPTER 9   The Universal Law of Attraction 50

CHAPTER 10   The Secret to Attracting Vibrant Health 54

APPENDIX A   Cutting-Edge Cancer Clinics & Resources 57

APPENDIX B   Recommended Readings, DVD's and Websites. 59

APPENDIX C   Vibrant Health Nutritional & Lifestyle Reference . . . 65

Cancer Research Archive 91
References 217

Acknowledgements

First of all, I would like to extend my gratitude toward the universal, creative source through which all life comes into being. The abundance and prosperity in all facets of my life have been the direct result of seeking understanding, along with becoming aligned with this perfect universal power. A naturally inquisitive soul, my life's ambition is driven by my quest to share the empowerment that knowledge provides with the world. I recognize my own power in co-creating my life and hope to share that with you, into whose hands this book has come.

A special offering of gratitude is passed on to the love of my life, Elizabeth, for her unwavering support in my endeavor to undertake this groundbreaking writing. Every day I am reminded of the fact she is the most remarkable person I have ever met. I am truly inspired by her love, intellect and comforting presence in my life. I would also like to thank my parents William and Virginia, my sisters Kayla and Kelli, my extended family, and friends for their tremendous support.

I must commend the following cutting-edge health pioneers and consumer advocates. These champions of information have taken investigative journalism to another level in order to expose the unethical and corrupt practices of many health industry giants.

- Joseph Mercola, DO
- Matthias Rath, MD
- Udo Erasmus, PhD
- Gary Null, PhD
- Kevin Trudeau
- Paul A. Goldberg, MPH, DC, DACBN
- John Donofrio, DC, DACNB
- Knox Grandison, DC
- Joe Thomas, D.C.

- William Shine, DC, DACNB

- Jeffrey Bland, PhD, FACN, CNS

These individuals seek to empower the public through knowledge. Our shared mission is to expose the erroneous and perpetually publicized corporate propaganda concerning health and medicine. I encourage you to support their remarkable efforts to change the face of healthcare as we know it.

INTRODUCTION

"All truth passes through three stages. First, it is ridiculed, second it is violently opposed, and third, it is accepted as self-evident."
—**Arthur Schopenhauer, Philosopher**

My intention in writing *Cracking the Cancer Code* is to create a quick, easy-to-understand and comprehensive reference to guide anyone diagnosed with cancer onto the path of empowerment and optimal health. Prosperity and abundance, in the form of health, indisputably manifests from the inside out.

In order to make *Cracking the Cancer Code* as reader-friendly as possible, I have divided the book into two primary sections. Part one begins by providing a brief overview of the nature, causes and common treatments of cancer. From this groundwork, I begin to elaborate on the various external and environmental factors that contribute to the development of the disease. This includes an emphasis on the tenets of proper, cutting-edge nutrition and an investigation into the environmental hazards that we unwittingly expose ourselves to on a daily basis. Part two of *Cracking the Cancer Code* centers on an examination of the internal environment—your thoughts, feelings and disposition—and the role it ultimately plays in your health. Throughout this groundbreaking work, the motif that I have intended to keep to the forefront is that the state of your health is entirely within your control.

Thanks to the pioneering efforts of modern quantum physics, it is now generally recognized that we, as human beings, are more than just the sum of our physical and tangible parts. Beyond the tissues, the organs or even the atoms that comprise our body we are all pure energy and vibrating particles. "Mind is movement and the body is the physical manifestation of that movement," philosopher Bob Proctor states. *Cracking the Cancer Code* examines the powerful implications of these facts.

Recognizing you, the reader, as the steward of your own body, my aim is to give you the tools and the encouragement to help you empower yourself to attain the extraordinary health that is waiting for you. The choice in how you receive this information—and how you decide to apply it to your own life—is ultimately yours. Whether you recognize it or not, you are already a co-creator of your own existence. As such, you have it within your power to change what you do not like and attract more of what you do. Take joy in learning how to better take care of yourself and becoming a more vital, energetic person. As you participate in *Cracking the Cancer Code*, know that there is no such thing as incurable.

PART I

1

CANCER AT A GLANCE

Incurable means curable from within. Disease is the body's way of giving you feedback that you are not loving or grateful.
—Dr. John Demartini

The National Cancer Institute estimates that one out of every two American men and women will develop some form of cancer during their lifetime. Cancer is *not* a mysterious illness that suddenly attacks out of the blue, rendering you helpless and powerless to something beyond your control. It has definite causes that are correctable if the human body has enough time to respond in order to counteract adverse changes occurring within the internal environment. This requires an alteration of the internal environment to one that creates health as opposed to cancer. Additionally, attacking the cancerous cells by taking advantage of their weaknesses can effectively be used as an adjunct therapy.

The word 'disease'—a term so often applied to the proliferation of cancerous cells—can be most simply understood to be a state of dis-ease or dis-comfort. *Taber's Cyclopedic Medical Dictionary* (19th Edition) defines disease as an unhealthy condition marked by subjective complaints, a specific history, and clinical signs, symptoms, and laboratory or radiographic findings. Dr. Wayne Dyer, however, provides a more expansive and empowering definition, boldly stating that disease "means the body is not in vibrational harmony (ease) with the creative source of the universe." The infinite universal power that permeates every atom and sub-particle of our existence is the ultimate source of vibrant health. A deeper comprehension of this concept is therefore critical when trying to understand and ultimately overcome an ailment like cancer. Before we begin to uncover the secrets of transforming your health from the inside out, let us quickly examine what cancer consists of from a medical perspective.

Cancer from a Medical Perspective

- Cancer is the general classification for over one hundred related medical conditions involving uncontrolled and dangerous cell growth.
- Cancer cells develop in the body as a result of damage to cellular DNA, which destroys the control mechanism of cell replication.[1]
- Scientists suggest that some cancer is caused by genetic factors.
- Scientists also suggest that *most* cancers are caused by environmental conditions.

In other words, one patient may already have a family history of breast cancer while another was exposed to a carcinogenic (cancer-causing) chemical in a factory. Both suffer from cancer. The difference between these two cases lies primarily in the underlying mechanism that initially triggered the abnormal cell growth. One of the most insidious aspects of cancer is the way it grows. As the tumor outgrows the original organ, pieces of malignant tissue often break off (metastasize) and invade the bloodstream or lymph system.[2] Cancer cells can then attach themselves to other vulnerable organs and start the formation of new tumors. Thus a patient with liver cancer may eventually suffer from lung, brain, or breast cancer as well. Approximately 90 percent of all cancer fatalities result from metastasis.

Traditional Medical Treatment

Conventional medical treatment for cancer generally fits into one of three categories: chemotherapy, radiation or surgical removal. Chemotherapy is defined by the American Cancer Society as the use of drugs for treating cancer. At its most basic, chemotherapy's short-term success depends on the ability to effectively poison and kill more cancerous cells than living cells. I make the statement that this is a short-term success because in several chemotherapy cases, patients will develop some form of secondary cancer as a result of exposure to such high levels of toxic chemicals. Similarly, radiation therapy—or the targeted bursts of radiation directed at cancerous tissues—carries a similar risk. Many radiation patients develop some form of secondary cancer within a few years of being declared "cancer free." The third approach to cancer treatment recognized in conventional medicine is surgery. Surgery, encompassing an invasion into the body and the physical removal of afflicted tissue, is rarely used on its own in the treatment of cancer. Rather, it is often accompanied by one of the aforementioned therapies as well. At is most simplified level, all these conventional treatments bring a certain level of risk and pain to the patient because they all operate on the same principal: destroy the cancer before the toxic chemicals and radiation destroy the host (you)!

Chemotherapy and Radiation

Chemotherapy utilizes powerful medicines, which claim to target and isolate the abnormally fast-growing cells. Unfortunately, this destruction also includes the disruption and sometimes cessation of normal body functions such as hair growth and digestion. Radiation treatments use heat energy to literally burn off malignant cells. Nevertheless, healthy tissue is also just as indiscriminately destroyed. Surgical removal can lead to a permanent recovery, but undetected malignant cells may have already metastasized to other organs or be jarred loose by surgical procedures.[3] Even when patients are able to survive such harsh medical therapies, the struggle for health often becomes continuous, as their weak bodies develop new illnesses or tumors.

A study completed in 1993 by German bio-statistician Ulrich Abel found that the overall success rate for most cancers treated with standard allopathic treatment (chemo, radiation, & surgery) was only **4 percent**. Statistically averaged, **96 percent** of cancer patients treated conventionally died of cancer or from complications related to their treatment. The only group of cancers treated conventionally that had a higher batting average was some blood cancers such as leukemia or Hodgkins, which approached a 35 percent success rate, still well below half.[4]

It was necessary to provide a little background on the conventional approach to cancer because, as you will see, the tone and the content of this book will not dwell on treating this disease—at least by the aforementioned means. Nor will it focus on the simple management of the common symptoms and side effects experienced by cancer patients. As I intend to demonstrate, treating the by-products (symptoms) of disease is a dead end pursuit. Ultimately, the treatment of any disease—cancer included—that centers around controlling or disguising the often painful symptoms without regard to the underlying cause will eventually fail. I state with 100 percent certainty that this is so because the symptoms, despite what you may think, are not the problem. It is the disruption in the body's natural tendency toward health that is the problem. Symptoms are merely an indicator of an underlying situation. Throughout the remainder of this book what I most want you to keep in mind is that, before all else, **cancer is the symptom and not the cause.**

Should you choose to be open to this power, you have the opportunity to attain extraordinary health. This book provides you with the knowledge that will enable you to empower yourself and allow your body to do what it was created to do. I am referring to the ability to begin the healing process from within.

In order for you to be able to focus on healing from within, I must first show you a new perspective concerning health and disease. My hope is that, empowered with such knowledge as I am able to impart, you will be able to change the way you choose to relate to your environment, your choices, your body and your role in your own state of health and well-being. Once you are able to change the way you look at things, you will be amazed at how quickly the things you look at change. Understanding the origins, history and private interests that historically shaped and continue to influence western medicine is essential to this process. Moreover, you must critically evaluate the prevalence of a symptom-based approach to treatment and its logical consequences. It is this issue that I will explore in the following chapters. With any luck, you will have a more thorough understanding of the foothold that sickness has on the American public and why the disease rates continue to climb.

2

THE BUSINESS OF HEALTHCARE

*"The art of medicine consists of amusing the patient
while nature cures the disease."*
—**Voltaire**

There are a number of alternative healing therapies that work so well and cost so little when compared to conventional treatment, that Organized Medicine, the Food & Drug Administration, and their overlords in the Pharmaceutical Industry (The Big Three) would rather the public not know about them. The reason is obvious: alternative, non-toxic therapies represent a potential loss of billions of dollars to allopathic medicine and drug companies.[1] Think this is too awful to be true? Read on.

The Big Three have collectively engaged in a medical collusion for over 70 years to influence legislative bodies at both the federal and state levels. The ultimate objective of which has been, and still is, to produce regulations that encourage the use of drug medicine while simultaneously creating restrictive, controlling mechanisms (licensing, government approval, etc) designed to limit and stifle the availability of non-drug, alternative modalities. The conspiracy to limit and eliminate competition from non-drug therapies began with the Flexner Report of 1910.

In 1910, Kentucky-born American educator Abraham Flexner was commissioned by oil tycoon John D. Rockefeller to tour the country and evaluate the effectiveness of therapies taught in medical schools and other institutions of the healing arts. History persuades us that Rockefeller, far from having altruistic intentions, wanted to dominate control over petroleum, petrochemicals and pharmaceuticals—which are all derived from coal tars or crude oil. He arranged for his company, Standard Oil of New Jersey to obtain a controlling interest in a huge German drug cartel called I. G. Farben. He was able to engage two of his stronger competitors, Andrew Carnegie of US Steel and JP Morgan of JP Morgan and Co. as partners, while making other, less powerful players, stockholders in Standard Oil. For these elite men, this consolidation of influential wealth enabled them to expand their power and control into the healthcare sector. Those who would not come into the fold were crushed according to a Rockefeller biographer.[2] Subsequently, during World War II Standard Oil of New Jersey was eventually accused of treason for this pre-war alliance with I.G. Farben.

The report Flexner submitted to The Carnegie Foundation was titled *Medical Education in the United States and Canada.* Expressed on page 22 of the report was the mandate: "the privileges of the medical school can no longer be open to casual strollers from the highway. It is necessary to install a *doorkeeper* who will, by critical scrutiny, ascertain the fitness of the applicant, a necessity suggested, in the first place, but consideration for the candidate, whose time and talents will serve him better in some other vocation, if he be unfit for this, and in the second, by consideration for a public entitled to protection from those whom the very boldness of modern medical strategy equips with instruments that, tremendously effective for good when rightly used, are all the more terrible for harm if ignorantly or incompetently employed."

As history has revealed, congress swallowed the recommendations of this report hook, line, and sinker. The end result, of course, has been to rob citizens of their freedoms in the name of public protection. It was decided that the American Medical Association (AMA), would be the doorkeeper. Not a bad idea, you may think. And you would be right, if that was all the AMA did. What I would like to bring your attention to is the fact that the AMA was now empowered to certify or de-certify any medical school in the country on the grounds of whether that school met the AMA's standards of *approved* medicine.[3]

Where the AMA really took the Flexner Report findings to heart lies in the still-present prejudice against alternative healing methods. Not surprisingly, Flexner found that any discipline that didn't use drugs to help cure the patient was tantamount to *quackery* and *charlatanism.* Here it is important to remember that John D. Rockefeller, who had huge stake in chemical giant I.G. Farben, commissioned Flexner to conduct this study. The argument may, therefore, be made that Flexner's findings were not wholly (or even partially) unbiased. As a result, medical schools that offered courses in bioelectric Medicine, Homeopathy or Eastern Medicine, for example, were told to either drop these courses from their curriculum or lose their accreditation and underwriting support. A few schools resisted for a time, but eventually most schools cooperated or were closed down. A similar scenario was played out in Canada. It was attempted in England against Homeopathy, but it failed due to the personal intervention of the Royal Family who had received much relief and healing at the hands of Homeopathic healers in the 19th century.[4]

The AMA came into existence in 1847. A private organization of allopathic physicians, it was originally formed to advance the interests of physicians, to promote public health, to lobby for medical legislation, and to raise money for medical education. The most important piece of information that I can hope to impart is that the AMA exists to serve the interests of its members. It functions in every sense of the word as a *union*, although its members wear white collars instead of blue. Nowhere is this more evident than in its ability to influence favorable legislation. Giving the AMA the power over the certification of medical schools is the equivalent of giving the Teamsters Union the exclusive right to decide on the laws of interstate commerce and transportation.[5] Is it any wonder that the total number of medical schools in the United States went from 160 in 1906 (before the Flexner Report) to 85 in 1920 and further down to 69 schools in 1944? A little like putting the fox in charge of the hen house, no?

Here in America, a relentless campaign of misinformation, fraud, deception, and suppression of alternative therapies and healers has been in place for the better part of this century. This has been done in order to keep highly effective alternative therapies from reaching any significant plateau of public awareness. Control is exerted through news items and propaganda from pro-establishment organizations like The AMA, The American Cancer Society, The Diabetes Foundation, etc.; local medical boards and government agencies like the FDA, The National Institute of Health (NIH), and The National Cancer Institute (NCI), The National Academy of Science, etc. All this is done, of course, with the full cooperation of the mainstream media which itself serves larger interests.[6] *The Doors of Perception* and *Expert Deception: PR Media Industry Exposed* are two incredible articles I've included within the research archive section of this work. They provide an in-depth investigation into the public relations industry and educate the reader on how to spot half-truths and propaganda.

Over the past decades, hundreds of caring, concerned, and conscientious alternative healers have been jailed and abused like common criminals for the so-called "crime" of curing people of life-threatening diseases in an unapproved manner. This has been carried out by heavy-handed government agents who swoop down on clinics with drawn guns, flax jackets, and Gestapo manners. All the while, these same agents and agencies behind this anti-alternative campaign posture themselves before TV cameras and the public under the ludicrous pretense of being servants of the people and protectors of the common good.[7] You may be shocked to find out that a federal judge found the AMA guilty of conspiracy to destroy the chiropractic profession in the 1987 Wilk case.

The medico-drug cartel was summed up by J.W Hodge, M.D., of Niagara Falls, N.Y., in these words: "The medical monopoly or medical trust, euphemistically called the American Medical Association, is not merely the meanest monopoly ever organized, but the most arrogant, dangerous and despotic organization which ever managed a free people in this or any other age. Any and all methods of healing the sick by means of safe, simple and natural remedies are sure to be assailed and denounced by the arrogant leaders of the AMA doctors' trust as fakes, frauds and humbugs Every practitioner of the healing art who does not ally himself with the medical trust is denounced as a 'dangerous quack' and impostor by the predatory trust doctors. Every sanitarian who attempts to restore the sick to a state of health by natural means without resort to the knife or poisonous drugs, disease imparting serums, deadly toxins or vaccines, is at once pounced upon by these medical tyrants and fanatics, bitterly denounced, vilified and persecuted to the fullest extent."[8] For more revelations about the origins of the business with disease, the AMA, the House of Rockefeller and the pharmaceutical industry read *Rockefeller Medicine Men* by E. Richard Brown and *The Drug Story* by Morris A. Bealle. An essay concerning the latter can be found in the research archive section of this work.

All too often, politicians are prepared to enact laws benefit the influential (moneyed) minority without regard to the impact that this may have on the less-aware public. It is no secret that the misuse, abuse and outright exploitation of funds in the political arena is an ongoing problem in politics. One need look no further than his or her daily newspaper for evidence. Unfortunately, despite the attention that is paid to the corrupt practices that riddle the American political scene, little lasting work has been done to correct the problem. At long last, however, the public's consciousness seems to have finally reached a critical mass and is now beginning to seriously question the efficacy and appropriateness of using ortho-dox therapies and allopathic medicine in general.[9]

I have included a historically accurate expose entitled, *The History of the Business with Disease* as the last piece of investigative research in the research archive section of this book. This will further acquaint you with the shocking history and evolution of modern medicine starting around WWII.

3

A NEW PERSPECTIVE ON HEALTH & DISEASE

The greatest mistake in the treatment of diseases is that there are physicians for the body and physicians for the soul, although the two cannot be separated.
—Plato

In the ever-changing world of orthodox allopathic medicine, there have been three things that have remained constant. These three concepts, in spite of major scientific breakthroughs in human nutrition, holistic/energy medicine and other alternative therapies—come from the very antiquated symptom-based paradigm. This approach places little emphasis on self-responsibility. This mentality of assigning accountability on external (and uncontrollable) factors—including genetic expression—is quickly losing its foothold on the American public's psyche. Below, I explore and rectify several common misconceptions regarding health and well being.

Misconception 1: Medicine and Allopathic physicians diagnose and treat symptoms in tandem disease using medications and surgical procedures to facilitate and restore health.

Consider this:

- Taber's Cyclopedic Medical Dictionary (19th Edition) states that *allopathy* is "a system of treating disease by inducing a pathological reaction that is antagonistic to the disease being treated." In layman's terms, this means **treating disease by using disease-producing reactions** (drugs, etc.). This confusing, illogical definition makes clear the reasons why traditional medical treatments are scientifically unable to permanently cure one single disease! In fact, the word 'cure'—as defined by the medical experts—has been corrupted and only refers to suppression of symptoms and is confined to a period of 1-5 years.

- Symptoms are not causative factors of underlying disease and are generally the last manifestation of illness. Covering them up with drugs and surgical removal of bodily tissue negates foundational knowledge that all of the systems in our physical body, work together like a finely tuned orchestra. This creative, universal force has designed our bodies perfectly! Here I refer not only to our physical beings, but to our emotional and spiritual beings as well.

- We are automatically equipped to heal ourselves. For example, have you ever had to tell a wound to heal, for the skin to knit itself together again? Have you ever even had to spend time consciously thinking about it? No, you have not. Your body has an innate tendency to achieve a healthful equilibrium. The medical term for this process is *homeostasis.* As I reveal the secrets to reconnecting with the body's internal healing capabilities, you will begin to experience amazing and abundant health as it was originally intended. Simply stated, *true health comes from within*!

Misconception 2: We are merely a physical being—only the sum of our tangible parts. Health, therefore, is only maintained and restored via external intervention. Treatment, in order to be effective, should only deal with that which can be empirically quantified. The spiritual, emotional and mental components of health, therefore, cannot be qualified.

Consider this:

- The universe operates around the principle of attraction. Essentially, the energy we send out—the thoughts we focus on—is the energy we attract to us. As we are in the age of enlightenment, mankind is becoming more aware that having a close spiritual connection with our Source (as Dr. Wayne Dyer states) allows our body's energy to resonate at a higher frequency to consequently manifest vibrant health! *Power versus Force* by David Hawkins, M.D., is based on over 25 years of scientific research on the impact our thoughts have on consciousness and muscle responses.

- The placebo effect, defined as the beneficial effect in a patient following a particular treatment that arises from the patient's expectations concerning the treatment rather than from the treatment itself, further refutes the misconception that your mental and emotional state does not have a significant impact on health and healing. In fact, in nearly half of all clinical trials of those patients in the control group (those receiving the placebo) experience some form of symptom relief.

Misconception 3: Bacteria, for the most part, are harmful for our body and consequently affect health in a negative manner. Anti-bacterial soaps, hand sanitizers, etc. are therefore helpful in maintaining health.

Consider this:

- Around 90 percent of all bacteria in and around your body are referred to as 'friendly bacteria' (probiotics) due to their beneficial effects. In fact, these very probiotics are responsible for supporting the healthy functioning of the digestive—and subsequently the immune—system. Sixty to eighty percent of the immune system can be found within the gut, thanks to these friendly microorganism inhabitants.

Exploring Germ Theory:

Pasteur's Germ Theory vs. Béchamp's Cellular Theory

The germ theory of disease, also called the pathogenic theory of medicine, is a theory that proposes that microorganisms are the cause of many diseases. Although not the first to suggest this theory, French microbiologist and chemist Louis Pasteur is often regarded as the father of germ theory for his work during the late 19th century. Although highly controversial when first introduced, it is now a cornerstone of modern conventional medicine and clinical microbiology. This theory was a theoretical foundation of epidemiology, the development and use of anti-microbial and antibiotic drugs, hygienic practices in hospitals, and public sanitation.

Germ theory has become the medical paradigm—the controlling medical idea—for the Western world. In its simplest form, germ theory proposes that the body is sterile and that germs from outside the body cause disease. Most of modern medical reaction to this theory has thus focused on developing the perfect drug to destroy these alien germs. No mainstream medical professional today does not subscribe to the germ theory.

Antione Béchamp, on the other hand, was a contemporary of Pasteur who maintained a pleomorphic theory, which was opposite the germ theory. Essentially

Béchamp's research showed bacteria change form and are *not the cause of*, but the *result of*, disease, arising from tissues rather than from a germ of constant form. This cellular disease theory holds that scavenging bacteria are supposed to arise from what he called microzymas (micro-organisms) that he says are present in matter (including tissues). These bacteria then feed on dead or decaying cells, or cells in need of repair. The bottom line is that *disease is built by unhealthy internal conditions.*[3]

The billion dollar pharmaceutical industry has taken away some of the symptoms and pain but has not found the answer for many infectious and most all degenerative diseases including cancer. Both the medical community and the individual must start examining what is causing the underlying illness in the first place. The cure then reveals itself.

As mentioned elsewhere throughout the text, self-responsibility and accountability has been rescinded. Many individuals subscribe to the notion that the solution lies beyond him- or herself. Rather, the cure is to be found in a pill, in chemotherapy, in radiation or in surgery. In short, the conventional medical community—aided and abetted by major media—has propagated a paradigm that most of America has blindly embraced for the last century: the drug is the cure. If germs from the air cause disease, the medical/pharmaceutical conglomerates must find the answer. Again, the individual is not responsible. What can we do to stop germs from the air getting in our mouths and our whole body? According to the germ theory, we can do nothing for a cure or to stop the cause of disease. There are always germs in the air. We are breathing in these germs right now. Some of us get sick and some of us do not get sick. For some of us who do get sick, the cold lingers for days. Others of us seem to get well very fast. It seems a more logical explanation is that germs are allowed to cause problems in our body when we do not have a strong immune system, enough good bacteria (dysbiosis), or healthy internal environment.[4] This, as I intend to show, is truly the case. The cure lies in a change of mind and a change of choice.

I'm *convinced*, based on my clinical expertise and extensive research into the cause of disease, Béchamp's cellular theory appears to be most plausible! As individuals seek to gain more knowledge and come to a higher state of awareness concerning health, the implications of what was just stated will resonate profoundly. Remember, there are millions of dollars generated by hanging onto Pasteur's flawed germ theory. Keeping the public sick and misinformed is good for the healthcare business.

The Ancient Origin of Western Medicine

To truly understand these previous misconceptions, the origin of western medicine and why they still thrive today, one has to be familiar with the ancient Greek schools of *Hygeia* and *Aesculapius*. The latter was the Greek god of medicine. The school that was named after him held the belief that toxic and invasive methods were required to suppress or treat symptoms, stop infections, cut body parts out or poison them in order to restore health. This form of thought evolved into modern day medicine that uses surgery (cutting), radiation (burning), and drug-oriented (poison) practices in an attempt to cure disease. Aesculapius' staff, with the snake coiled around it, is the symbol of medicine and the official emblem of the American Medical Association.[1]

Hygeia, on the other hand, was the Greek goddess of health and beauty. Today, this would be considered the natural, holistic approach to healing. The entire concept of this treatment was to place the body in harmony with nature to construct, rebuild, and strengthen the body so that infections could not take hold. The second goal was to increase the innate resistance to infection and deterioration. Lastly, the objective was to raise and support the body's natural healing mechanisms with the use of natural substances if infection or deterioration was present. The school of Hygeia recognized that healing took place from within and sought to provide the body with the tools it needed to innately heal itself. The focus was on proper nutrition, clean water, fresh air, sunlight, healing touch, herbs, physical activity, massage, love, and other natural, non-invasive methods.[2]

Historically, these lines of thought actually have their beginnings about 2200 years before Hippocrates (Western Father of Medicine) and the Greeks. Imhotep, a famous ancient Egyptian doctor, was the first apparent figure of a physician to stand out clearly from the mists of antiquity!

Examining Internal and External Toxicity

Most healers agree that any influence that depresses the functional capacity of our liver elevates our risk of cancer. Total load refers to the *total of all exposures* and influences that bear on human physiology (how the body functions). [5] In other words, everything, when taken collectively, that impacts the functioning of the human body. When we *insult* our bodies with unclean water, polluted air, toxins (pesticides, alcohol, cigarettes, heavy metals), drugs (antibiotics, aspirin etc.), improper nutrition, food additives/dyes, stress, and other lifestyle factors, our liver and gastrointestinal tracts break down. Over time the functional capacity of these organs becomes severely decreased, which consequently inhibits their ability to detoxify and process the barrage of *toxic garbage* coming in. We then start to suffer the effects of toxic *overload,* which manifest as chronic disease processes. A periodic detoxification regimen in the form of *fasting* is absolutely necessary to prevent this from happening.

On a side note, I encourage you to reference the **APPENDIX C** section I've included in this book. All of the food and household products that are recommended will help to *significantly reduce the total load on your body!*

Garbage In, Garbage Out

In 1900 only one in seven people died of cardiovascular disease, and only one in thirty people died of cancer. Today, those figures have grown to 1 in 3 and 1 in 2, respectively. Between that time and today, something basic and critical to health has changed. This span of history includes *processed foods* becoming a mega-industry; the introduction of *pesticides*; the rising of *pharmaceutical drugs*; increased *industrial pollution* of the soil, water, and air; *chlorination* of water; *car exhaust; tobacco smoke;* indoor pollution through the use of *synthetic chemicals* for everything—cleaners, body-care and make-up, paints, carpets, and furniture.[6] All of these things I've mentioned severely *weaken* the immune system and alter the internal environment within the body. Thus, creating the ideal conditions for the development and growth of cancer.

Now that we've unearthed a different perspective and cleared up a few misconceptions concerning the notions of health mentioned above, I intend to investigate the nutritional essentials of health and healing. This will allow a greater understanding of how encompassing and important the process of nourishing the body truly is. Proper nutrition sets the stage for the body to be the *true doctor* and heal itself! Remember:

- The power that made the body heals the body!

4

THE STANDARD AMERICAN DIET (SAD)

"The doctor of the future will give no medicine but will interest his patients in the care of the human frame, in diet and in the cause and prevention of disease."
—Thomas Edison

The Standard American Diet (SAD) has become a staple of what most individuals in this country consume on a regular basis. This toxic diet consists of processed foods (not limited to fast-food), low fiber content and hydrogenated fats, refined carbohydrates, artificial sweeteners, and additives. The SAD that was just described is simply a result of becoming out of touch with nature and allowing private interest groups to think for us!

- In 1815 sugar consumption was fifteen pounds per person per year. Today it stands at one hundred thirty-five pounds per person per year. Cardiovascular disease (CVD), diabetes, and obesity result from increased use of refined sugars, refined starches, and calorie-rich foods. In the 1800's, CVD deaths were extremely rare. They rose to one in seven deaths by 1900, and today account for more than one death in every three.[1]

- Diabetes rose at a similar rate and, if one includes cardiovascular complications, now accounts for one death in twenty. About thirty percent of adults in Western society are obese, risking cancer, CDV, diabetes, allergies, and a whole host of other degenerative ailments.[2]

Meat Production

The commercialization of meat production illustrates most clearly how taking control of our food supply (domesticating, breeding, and artificial feeding) has affected its nutritional content and our physical health. Today, much of the cattle in the U.S. does not graze on green pastures and are not allowed to roam free, like portrayed on the product labels. Instead most live their lives on feeding lots *confined* to small areas and are fed grain, as opposed to their natural diet of grass. The grain is what gives steak the fatty, marble look. This drastically elevates the saturated fat and cholesterol content within the meat and dairy (milk, cheese, yogurt, etc).

Most cattle in the United States (unless certified organic) are injected with Bovine Growth Hormone (BGH), fed antibiotics, and then the feed lots are blanketed with insecticides which fall into the cattle's food and water and eventually become part of someone's dinner. *The cattlemen found that when they inject BGH into a cow it produced between 15-25% more milk* although it seriously damaged the animal's health and reproduction capacity. This injected hormone significantly increased their profit margin however this is terrible news for you and especially children. We note that kids today are physically maturing at an unusually earlier age now. I'm convinced based on widespread expert research there is an obvious and direct correlation between conventional food production, early physical maturation, and reproductive organ cancers. This would explain the fact that every industrialized country in the world, except for the US, has banned BGH! I've included an article entitled *Milk and the Cancer Connection* in the Research Archive section of this work which exposes the link between cancer and BGH in greater depth.

When the animal products mentioned above are ingested, you are also indirectly flooding your system with synthetic antibiotics. *Bearing in mind that 90 percent of the bacteria in and around your body are beneficial and vital to your overall health, antibiotics are unable discriminate between good and bad bacteria.* They kill everything! Vast quantities of certain antibiotics are routinely included in the diet of healthy farm animals because this practice has been shown to make animals grow faster. Experts have recently concluded this ultimately leads to an environment conducive to the evolution of antibiotic resistance.

Poultry is produced and processed in a similar fashion. Chickens are possibly the most abused animal on the face of the planet. Conventional chickens are crammed in filthy sheds by the tens of thousands, immersed in their own excrement among the corpses of other birds who died of heart attacks or stress. Some even die of starvation by becoming crippled from growing so large, so fast, that their legs cannot withstand the weight which makes them unable to reach food. The birds are genetically manipulated then fed antibiotics to produce unnatural rapid growth. This usually results in their hearts, lungs, and legs breaking down under the added weight. Unquestionably, these birds endure a very cruel, unsanitary environment. The chickens are then forced to have their beaks clipped so they can't peck at each other and risk infection. Lastly, they are given growth hormones to make them mature much faster so the corporations can boost their bottom line quicker. *Diet for a New America* by John Robbins does a great job at investigating and exposing the brutality of non-organic food manufacturing. Routine cruelty is the cold, inescapable reality for animals raised on modern conventional production farms that eventually are killed in slaughterhouses across the country.

Milk Pasteurization and Homogenization

The process of milk pasteurization destroys valuable enzymes, decreases vitamin content, denatures fragile milk proteins, destroys vitamins B12, B6, and C, kills beneficial bacteria, promotes pathogenic bacteria growth and is linked with allergies. Pasteurization also promotes accelerated tooth decay, colic in infants, growth problems in children, osteoporosis, arthritis, heart disease and cancer. Calves that are fed pasteurized milk do poorly and many die before maturity. Homogenization is thought, by many experts, to be a leading causative factor in heart disease due to research that suggests this process induces scaring of the arteries.

Raw milk sours naturally but pasteurized milk turns putrid; processors must remove slime and pus from pasteurized milk by a process of centrifugal clarification. Inspection of dairy herds for disease is not required for pasteurized milk. Pasteurization was instituted in the 1920s to combat TB, infant diarrhea, undulant fever and other diseases caused by poor animal nutrition and dirty production methods. But times have changed and modern stainless steel tanks, milking machines, refrigerated trucks and inspection methods make pasteurization absolutely unnecessary for public protection.[3]

Pasteurization does not always kill the bacteria for Johne's disease suspected of causing Crohn's disease in humans with which most confined cows are infected.[4]

Most commercial milk is now ultra-pasteurized to get rid of heat-resistant bacteria and give it a longer shelf life. Ultra-pasteurization is a violent process that takes milk from a chilled temperature, to above the boiling point in under two seconds. Clean raw milk (unpasteurized and non-homogenized) from certified healthy cows is available commercially in several states and may be bought directly from the farm in many more. (Sources are listed on www.realmilk.com.)

Pesticides and Herbicides

The majority of the produce (not labeled organic) found in conventional grocery stores, contain some type of pesticide, insecticide, or fungicide. Would you spray the bug killer Raid on your vegetables and fruits? When you buy food in boxes, cans, jars, fruits and vegetables that are not 100 percent organic, they have all been sprayed with deadly pesticides, fungicides, and herbicides which are ten to one hundred times more powerful than Raid! [5] What is truly frightening is that many of these pesticides have never been studied in great detail due to effective lobbying by the food industry! One would think that the FDA would mandate this because they are supposedly looking out for our best interest. However, the following quote by Herbert Lay (former FDA commissioner) says it best. He has stated *"What the FDA is doing and what the public thinks its doing are as different as night and day!"*

The notion that you can now just wash pesticides and herbicides off of your fruits and vegetables is, for the most part, wishful thinking. After the initial harvest, the pesticides can seep into the soil and eventually become absorbed by the roots and seeds of the plants. These poisons are now able to alter the genetic make-up of the plant and now become part of the DNA. This has major implications as far as health and healing are concerned. If you have not done so already, it would be wise to start investing in *organic* produce.

Genetically Modified Foods (GMO's)

Soy, potatoes, corn, and canola oil are some of the major products to be genetically modified these days. If the label does not say organic/non-GMO somewhere on it, move on to produce and oils that do. GMO's can wreak havoc on the immune system and internal organ integrity. Monsanto's director of corporate communications was quoted October 25, 1998 in The New York Times stating, "Monsanto should not have to vouchsafe the safety of biotech food. Our interest is in selling as much of it as possible. Assuring its safety is the FDA's job." This blatant disregard for consumer safety and shuffling responsibility by this corporate giant is yet another reason to start educating and empowering yourself when it comes to protecting your health.

Many have stated the entire GMO movement was brought about to meet the demand for the massive, ever-growing world population. While I agree that starvation and malnutrition are very real problems, they are precipitated by unequal distribution of wealth, not by food scarcity. According to the United Nations World Food Program, there is currently more than enough food produced to feed everyone on the planet an adequate and healthy diet. The reason that approximately 800 million people go hungry each year is that they don't have access to food by either being able to afford it or grow their own. Biotechnology, by turning living crops into intellectual property, increases corporate control over food resources and production. Rather than alleviate world hunger, biotechnology is likely to exacerbate it by increasing everybody's dependence on the corporate sector for seeds and the materials. Ronnie Cummins outlines the numerous health hazards of GMO's in his informative book entitled *Genetically Engineered Food*. 'Franken-Foods' will never be as perfect for the body as *real* living foods from the earth as given by our Universal Source.

In continuing with the subject of genetic modification, it would also be a good idea to eliminate your microwave oven. Exhaustive research from the Soviet Union concluded microwaves can cause cancer, decrease food value (bioavailability), and exert unpredictable negative effects upon the general biological welfare of humans! These are the primary factors that contributed to the Soviet's ban on microwave oven use in 1976. Nuking of food is also known to produce genetically altered proteins called prions, whose effects are currently being studied in great detail. See *The Hidden Hazards of Microwave Cooking* by Anthony Wayne and Lawrence Newell. Convection ovens are superior, quickly heat up food, and can be used as a microwave replacements. See **APPENDIX C** for the oven I recommend.

5

PUBLIC HEALTH HAZARDS EXPOSED

"Every human being is the author of his own health or disease."
—**Buddha**

Electromagnetic Pollution

Throughout the world today, there is a new form of pollution that has to be addressed when we discuss the road to vibrant health. This exposure that I'm referring to is Electromagnetic radiation. Radiation in this form is produced by anything that has an electrical current passing through it! Investigative research performed over the past twenty years imply possible connections of electromagnetic fields (EMF's) with brain cancer, miscarriages, birth defects, leukemia, breast cancer, and lymphomas. Practically everywhere you go you bump into EMF's from:

- Cell phones
- Power lines
- Satellites and Radar
- Microwave ovens
- Computers, television sets, alarm clocks
- Fluorescent lights
- Local media transmission towers
- Hair dryers,

- X-ray's, CAT scans, MRI (potentially deadly if used indiscriminately)

A great deal of EMF exposure can be curtailed or avoided since it occurs in the average home through electric blankets, computers, television sets, microwave ovens, and hair dryers. I recommend keeping your distance from these devices while in use. Make use of regular blankets instead of electrical ones. Double check all appliances and electrical installations in your home, making sure they are in working order with all protective devices and protocols in place. To accurately measure the amount of electromagnetic pollution coming from electrical devices along with different areas of the home, purchase a TriField™ Meter. This is the only EMF meter which offers magnetic, electric, and radio/microwave detection in one package (http://www.trifield.com/).

Chlorination

Remember, 90 percent of the bacteria in and around your body are vitally beneficial and necessary for you. Chlorine, like antibiotics, destroys the good bacteria in your gut when chlorinated water is taken in through unfiltered drinking water. Chlorine can also be credited for:

- Eating through lead pipes
- Corroding many types of metals
- Harming cells and DNA of every living organism it comes into contact with

Chlorine also introduces to our water supply some highly carcinogenic chemicals called trihalomethanes (THM's). Studies show a strong link between chlorinated water supplies with elevated THM levels and cancers of the bladder, kidney, liver, pancreas, GI tract, urinary tract, colon, and brain.[1]

Beneficial bacteria are compromised when this water comes in contact with your skin, let alone the toxic vapors that arise in a hot, chlorinated shower. I recommend using a chlorine shower filter. In the back of this book (**APPENDIX C**) I have listed some useful products and companies that I use on a regular basis. For a long list of published research/history of damaging effects of chlorine, visit www.mercola.com or www.garynull.com and key in chlorination in the search engine. Joseph Mercola, D.O. and Gary Null, PhD have the largest online research archives in the world. Their investigative research and documentation are impeccable.

Fluoridation

Fluoride is a substance that's highly poisonous, particularly in the salt-based form added in mouthwash and toothpaste. Moreover, its effectiveness is questionable at best. A top Environmental Protection Agency (EPA) scientific advisor voiced the opinion that "since recent federal government tests have shown that fluoride appears to cause cancers at levels less than ten times the present maximum contamination level, this would ordinarily require that all additions of fluoride water supplies be suspended and treatment be instituted to remove naturally occurring fluoride."[2] In my opinion, that should've immediately raised a red flag! (On a side note, I haven't come across any evidence that the EPA ever postponed the fluoridation process). I recommend choosing non-fluoridated alternatives for oral hygiene just to be on the safe side.

Fluoride has been connected to many different kinds of physiological problems. In my expert analysis, the most notable is hypothyroidism. This is a condition where the thyroid gland becomes under active and its ability to function correctly is compromised. If the thyroid gland is not functioning efficiently, your metabolism becomes incredibly slow, allowing you to easily gain weight. It has been suggested that fluoride in toothpaste and drinking water is one of the primary reasons why we have such high *hypothyroidism* and *obesity* rates in America today. Additionally, the United States is one of the only countries in the world to add fluoride to water.

Plastics, Food Wraps, and Drinking Bottles

Plastic products leach cancer causing toxins into our food supply. The toxicity is elevated when foods include large amounts of water or when they are extremely acidic. Water is one of nature's most effective solvents, and it is effective at drawing out toxins from plastic. The *Safe Shopper's Bible* states cling film contains carcinogenic by-products such as di-2-ethylhexyl phthalate (DEHP) and di-2-ethylhexyl (adipate) (DEHA), while plastic wrap contains residual traces of vinylidene chloride.[3] Aluminum wrap is not a great alternative either because it is well understood that it's harmful. A small quantity of aluminum inevitably permeates into foods it comes into contact with.

If you wash and reuse plastic water bottles, be aware that researchers say repeated washing and reuse of disposable water bottles may accelerate the breakdown of the plastic, increasing your exposure to potentially harmful chemicals.[4] I recommend when using water containers to use grade seven or above. On most water containers, you will see a triangle with a number inside when you flip the bottle upside-down. Anything less than grade seven is a sure-shot you're consuming the oil derived byproducts that have been released into the bottled drinking water.

Teflon

Teflon™ has been in the news quite a bit in the last year because Teflon™ nonstick pans have been shown to be extremely dangerous according to recent studies. When Teflon™ is heated at high temperatures, noxious fumes are produced that are poisonous to the human body. The Associated Press reports that a five billion class action lawsuit is being filed against Dupont, stating that the chemical giant failed to warn consumers of the dangers of a Teflon chemical.[5] The various chemicals that are used in manufacturing Teflon™ products have been linked to cancer by an overwhelming amount of research. It is postulated that this company has known for over twenty years that Teflon™ was linked to cancer and has suppressed this information for the sake of increasing their bottom line.[6] This possible cover-up illustrates another appalling example of a major corporation committing crimes against humanity for the sake of profit. If you own non-stick cookware, I recommend getting rid of it ASAP.

Deodorants and Antiperspirants

Many of us are familiar with the dangers of antiperspirants, and now recent scientific studies are elevating awareness about toxic effects of deodorants as well. Deodorants and antiperspirants are two slightly different entities. Deodorants operate by neutralizing the smell of the sweat and by antibacterial action against germs, but do not stop sweating. Antiperspirants operate by congesting or blocking the pores that discharge sweat (the active ingredient being aluminum) so that they can't release sweat. The apprehension with antiperspirant use is that the aluminum it contains is absorbed by the body and causes chaos in the brain, where it possibly contributes to the increasing numbers of individuals falling ill with Alzheimer's disease. Antiperspirants have also been acknowledged as a possible major cause in the development of breast cancer.

Dr. Kris McGrath, an allergist in Chicago who says he has found a correlation between antiperspirants, underarm shaving and cancer, conducted an investigative study in 2004. Dr. McGrath is convinced the culprits in antiperspirants are the toxins in aluminum salts like aluminum chlorohydrate. He has stated they don't generally infiltrate the skin enough to create problems, unless the skin is shaven. Disrupting the skin by shaving can make the body susceptible, because beneath the skin is the lymphatic system, which is attached to the breast tissue.

Recently, British scientific experts found traces of paraben chemicals in breast tissue samples taken from women with breast cancer. Researches also published a study not so long ago in the Journal of Toxicology that implied cosmetics applied underarm may be a causative factor in the development of breast cancer (study included in the Research Archive section). I recommend using organic deodorants or the Thai crystal deodorant stone. These do not contain any synthetic chemicals like parabens or propylene glycol. Be sure to read the labels because all natural deodorants are not paraben-free. On the deodorant labels avoid anything that contains methyl paraben, ethyl paraben, propyl paraben, butyl paraben, isobutyl paraben and E216.

6

MODERN SOCIETY PAYS A HEAVY PRICE

"I believe that there is a subtle magnetism in Nature, which, if we unconsciously yield to it, will direct us aright."
—Henry David Thoreau

Author and researcher Michael T. Murray, N.D., has elaborated in great detail about the absence of present-day disease from ancient cultures. He concluded that a number of aboriginal, primitive societies in Australia, Africa, and South America successfully passed into the twentieth century and enjoyed remarkably low rates of cancer, rheumatoid arthritis, obesity, diabetes, osteoporosis, heart disease, and other "modern" conditions *until they switched to modern diets*.[1]

Modern civilization has managed to infiltrate the culture of many of these once-isolated societies. Few of them still consume the primitive, simple diets of their ancestors. American travelers are often surprised to find that canned Western-style food, refined sugar, and white flour products are now consumed nearly everywhere in the world. As one might expect, this transition from primitive diets to modern diets has brought *deadly consequences*.[2]

The Astonishing Discovery of Albert Schweitzer

Albert Schweitzer has long been recognized for his pioneering international contributions to cancer prevention. In 1913, the Nobel Prize-winning physician visited Garbon, Africa and stated the following:

- "I was astonished to encounter no cases of cancer. I saw none among the natives two hundred miles from the coast.... I cannot, of course, say posi-

28

tively that there was no cancer at all, but like other frontier doctors, I can only say that, if any cases existed they must have been quite rare. This absence of cancer seemed to be due to the difference in nutrition of the natives compared to the Europeans."[3]

An Amazing Finding Among the Inuit

Vilhjalmur Stefansson was an explorer and anthropologist who searched endlessly for cases of cancer among the Inuit population while exploring the Arctic. Meticulous diary entries of his experiences and observations appear throughout his book *Cancer: Disease of Civilization*. Stefansson said a whaling ship doctor named George B. Leavitt found only *one cancer case in forty-nine years* among the Inuit of Alaska and Canada.[4] By the 1970's though, breast cancer malignancy appeared frequently among the Inuit women *after they began consuming a modern diet*. Toxic chemicals from our modern foods and industries have, without a doubt contributed to the condition.[5]

In today's society, roughly 90 percent of what you encounter at traditional grocery stores should not be classified as food! Modern supermarket food is devitalized due to contaminants and processing by food manufacturers. These substances do not nourish the body and are far from health promoting. *There is great news, though!* As people have begun to empower themselves, become more health conscious, and realize the body's health is directly related to what you put into it, the demand has increased considerably for real, organic living foods. Modern, cutting-edge grocers like Whole Foods Market, Wild Oats Market, and smaller organic grocers are flourishing, forcing the other mainstream, antiquated supermarkets to carry more organic products.

7

THE ESSENTIALS OF
HEALTH AND HEALING

"You are not nourished by the food you eat, but in proportion to the amount
you digest and assimilate."
—Herbert Shelton

When examining the essentials of health and healing, it is imperative to have an all-inclusive understanding of the entire nutritional process occurring in the human body. Let me begin by providing the appropriate definition of nutrition. *Nutrition* is the sum of all the processes involved in transforming, food, air, and water into living animated tissues, as Dr. Paul Goldberg writes in *Hygienic Heights.*[1] Many times the term nutrition is incorrectly applied to only the intake of food into the human body. From the biochemical and gastrological perspective, the five processes involved in the conversion of food to living tissues (after a supply of nutrients is ingested) are as follows:

- **Digestion**—occurs in the stomach and small intestine and requires cooperation from the liver and pancreas to break down food into water and fat-soluble molecules.[2]

- **Absorption**—occurs when food and nutrients are taken through the intestinal lining the bloodstream, and to the portal vein to the liver where it is filtered. From the bloodstream it passes to the cells. Until food is absorbed, it is essentially outside the body, in a tube going through it.[3]

- **Assimilation**—resourcefully shuttling the nutrients from the blood and lymphatic system into individual cells.

- **Excretion**—the method of getting rid of waste from the cell and doing so efficiently.

- **Elimination**—refers to the process of removing wastes effectively from the body through the kidneys, bowels, lymph system, and skin.

I am convinced the 10 ESSENTIALS OF HEALTH AND HEALING are as follows, based upon my extensive research and knowledge of the human body.

1. Strong Spiritual Connection to the Universal Intelligence

2. Positive Mental Attitude (Love, Happiness, Gratitude, Laughter, Optimism)

3. Nourishment (Organic, living foods and correcting Nutritional deficiencies)

4. Freedom from Toxic Influences, Emotions, and Chemicals

5. Water (reverse osmosis)

6. Sunlight

7. Oxygen

8. Physical Activity

9. Sleep and Rest

10. Fasting

Optimizing your Health Nutritionally

Following the traditional vague advice which recommends eating your fruits and vegetables, is *not* conducive to the pursuit of optimal health from a nutritional perspective. The quality of the food source and farming practices are rarely made relevant when you listen to supposed experts in the mainstream media. This is an ongoing problem because the quality of the food source and farming practices are, by a long-shot, *the most significant* aspects to consider when selecting food! One of my primary recommendations is to consume fresh, unprocessed foods focusing on natural, organic plant foods with additional amounts of lightly cooked plant foods. Most diets should consist primarily of:

- Organic fruits and vegetables
- Organic nuts and seeds
- Organic legumes and whole grains (minimal)

- Modest amounts of animal proteins such as organic, free-range eggs, chicken (free range/antibiotic and hormone free), fresh water (not farm raised) fish like salmon, halibut, mackerel, sardines and rainbow trout, as well as occasional organic, *grass-fed* red meat if desired. Pork can be excluded completely since it is devoid of nutritional benefits and many health risks are associated with its consumption.

Make *absolutely sure* the fish are tested for metal contaminants wherever you purchase.

All of these products should be in the ORGANIC form to ensure superior nutrition. Organic, fresh, raw foods possess forms of energy not currently understood by orthodox science. Organic produce is also higher in nutrient density than conventional produce. Basically, this is because of the farming practices associated. Organic farmers rotate their crops more frequently than do conventional farmers. This crop rotation dramatically affects the nutrient density of the food due to the fact that the soil has a longer period of time to replenish the nutrients it holds. Labels should specify one hundred percent organic should contain the word organic before each of the ingredients!

As far as name brand food products are concerned, I recommend avoiding them altogether. This is because they are publicly traded corporations that have been a part of deceptive misinformation campaigns by the food industry for years. These corporations spend millions of dollars lobbying each year in order to have their products classified as safe and all natural when that couldn't be farther from the truth! Please review the recommended texts and websites section of my book as this will give you an invaluable source on your journey of self-empowerment.

Avoid these Products Completely

Refined Carbohydrates—These consist of refined *sugar* and *starches* and foods that contain them. Examples of these are found in breads, pastas, and many products listed below. Many times you will see "enriched or bleached" white or wheat flower, high-fructose corn syrup, dextrose, and multidextrin, on the food labels. These types of foods upset and unbalance the body's chemistry due to their depleted nutritional value and harmful chemical constituents. For example, since the outer coating is stripped from the sugar/starch during the refining process, our body has to draw upon its own enzymes and mineral supply to digest them.[4] The human body is constantly functioning at a deficit due to these processed foods. There are numerous research studies that show decreases in immune function following refined sugar consumption. Subsequently, refined sugar consumption promotes an acidic environment within the body, wreaks havoc on the immune system, and *feeds* cancer cells! See *Cancer's Sweet Tooth* in the cancer research archive section of this book.

Packaged and junk foods (calorie—rich foods) including fast food, soda pop/soft drinks, fruit juices and drinks, candy, cake, white bread, white sugar (all of the previous are classified as *refined carbohydrates*), coffee, tea, commercial cow's milk, alcohol, or other junk food products. A good rule of thumb is, "if it isn't found in nature then don't allow yourself to eat it."

Saturated Fat Consumption—

Let me start by saying all saturated fat is not bad like many have been led to believe. Food production, processing, and preparation determine the integrity of the fat. The association between fats—meaning most saturated fats, rancid fats, refined omega 6's, and processed oils—and cancer has long been documented. I recommend avoiding the obvious and hidden sources of fat listed below.

- *Obvious Sources* of poor-quality fat such as margarines, shortenings, and butter. Limit refined vegetable oils and discard visible fats on beef, lamb, and pork, and the skin on chicken or turkey.[5]

- *Hidden Sources* of saturated fat are abundant in land-based, animal products that have been *grain-fed* (*red meat* [beef, pork, lamb], *dairy* [cheeses, cows milk, yogurt, conventional eggs], etc.) Avoid processed foods containing hidden fats, such as sausage, greasy burgers, fried foods, potato chips, and oily salad dressings.[6]

Altered Fats have been linked to cancer, atherosclerosis, mutations, and degeneration of cells, tissues and organs. The main sources are hydrogenated oil products. These include shortenings, margarines (hard and soft), shortening oils, deep-fried oils, and partially hydrogenated vegetable oils (used in convenience, processed, and junk foods). They are also found in bakery products, candies, French fries, fried and deep fried foods, and processed convenience foods and snacks such as potato and corn chips and other bagged snacks.[7]

Free-radicals are extremely reactive and unstable chemical species that have a single unpaired electron in an outer orbital.[8] Free-radicals are found in foods that are overcooked (browned/blackened). They are combated by having a diet high in Antioxidants (Vitamins A, C, E, along with Zinc, and Selenium), which are found in abundance in fruits, vegetables, nuts and seeds.

Sweeteners (Artificial & Natural)

- *Aspartame*™ (found in *Nutrasweet*™ products and *diet sodas*) contains aspartic acid in it and breaks down to formaldehyde in the body, hence is extremely toxic.[9] Formaldehyde is what morticians use to embalm the recently deceased. It is also an excitatory toxin (see below). Famed scientist, Morando Soffritti, has extensively studied Aspartame™ and concluded that it causes cancer! *Neotame*™ is an aspartame derivative that has the same effects.

- *Saccharin*™, and *Acesulfame K*™ (*Sunette*™/*Sweet One*™/*Sweet'N Low*™ products) have been studied and shown to have carcinogenic effects.[10]

- *Sucralose*, which is found in the popular sugar replacement *Splenda*™, is an excitatory toxin that is 600 times sweeter than sucrose (table sugar). One small study of diabetic patients using the sweetener showed a statistically significant increase in glycosylated hemoglobin, which is a marker of long-term blood glucose levels and is used to assess glycemic control in diabetic patients.[11] According to the FDA, "increases in glycosolation (huge amounts of sugar packed around the hemoglobin molecule) in hemoglobin imply lessening of control of diabetes." This is bad news in the short and long run. Some of the more common products *Splenda*™ is found in are foods, beverages, cold remedies, vitamins, and is now expanding to pharmaceuticals.

Additives and Colorings—I recommend staying away from food additives along with dyes due to their poisonous effect on the body. MSG (monosodium glutamate, glutamic acid, hydrolyzed protein) is a known excitatory toxin to neurons (brain and nerve cells) within the human body. When MSG is ingested, it causes an over-stimulatory effect on the neurons, killing many and severely fatiguing others.[12] This is what gives you a sensation of fullness. Many buffet restaurants still use MSG to prevent you from eating all the food! *Excitotoxins* by Russell Blaylock provides an in-depth, scientific exploration of the detrimental effects of MSG and Aspartame.

*Brand Name Cosmetics, Skin-care, Toothpastes, Soaps, Detergents, Shampoos, Etc…*These products are regularly produced with chemicals that have been heavily researched and found to be cancer causing! They also harm the skin by destroying its natural pH. Scrutinize every product label very carefully and don't buy products with the following chemicals contained in them.

- Propylene Glycol—main ingredient in anti-freeze and used in hydraulic fluids.

- Diethanolamine (DEA)—used as a wetting agent in shampoos, lotions, creams and other cosmetics.

- Sodium Lauryl Sulfate—used in shampoos, soaps, detergents, and tooth-pastes and other products that we expect to "foam-up."

- Hexachlorophene—used in soaps, deodorants, and cosmetics.

- Parabens—used primarily in skin-care products. Recent evidence indi-cates that topical parabens have been detected in human breast tumors. This is of great concern as parabens have been shown to mimic the action of the female hormone estrogen, which can encourage the growth of human breast tumors.

- Triclosan—found in most antibacterial soaps and may pose a threat to the liver.

- Any synthetic chemical at all. If you can't pronounce it, stay away!

Kevin Trudeau makes a great point as he has stated several times, "If you can't eat it, you shouldn't put it on your skin!" The skin is the largest organ of the body and absorbs much of the toxic chemicals that are applied to it. If you're not con-vinced, try this experiment at home. Mince some garlic at home and either place it in the palms of your hand or on the soles of your feet and I promise you will have garlic breath within twenty minutes!

The Safe Shopper's Bible written by Samuel Epstein, MD, is an excellent reference for anyone concerned about the health effects of ingredients in the items they buy every day—from soup to flea powder, mascara, or car wax. *The Safe Shopper's Bible* is truly indispensable.

Nutritional Recommendations

Drink ONLY reverse osmosis filtered water. Distilled water can be consumed mini-mally as well. These types of water are pure and more importantly do not contain chlorine and many other contaminants! *Distilled water collects and removes miner-als that have been rejected by the cells of the body and are therefore nothing more than debris, obstructing the normal functions of the system.* We should eat *living foods* and drink pure water. Living foods resonate at higher frequencies and therefore are able to transfer *energy* to our bodies. Water, is the only true drink! Products such as coffee, soda, and alcohol should be in the category of drugs, as opposed to foods. I recommend discontinuing them from the dietary regimen *permanently*.

Chew thoroughly, eating only when hungry in a relaxed, unhurried environment. Far too often people see eating as something that can be performed while engaging in numerous other tasks simultaneously (watching TV, driving in the car, etc.). When you eat under *stressful conditions*, your body will not efficiently digest and assimilate the food that comes in.

Ingest ONLY raw and slightly cooked foods because the nutrients are preserved best in those states! This rule is applicable to vegetables, fruits, nuts, and seeds. Some vegetables may be steamed and some grains need to be cooked as well

Consume Healing Fats. The healing fats in cancer include essential fatty acids (EFA's) and fresh, unrefined oils that contain them. EFA's, especially omega 3's, enhance oxygen use in cells, decrease tumor formation, slow tumor growth, decrease the spread of cancer cells (metastasis), and extend the survival time.[13]

Do not eat to the point of feeling full. This is considered overeating and actually places more stress on the gut.

Steaming, baking, or broiling in stainless steel (waterless) cookware are preferable ways to cook food. This cookware will not leach harmful chemicals into your system when preparing food at high temperatures like Teflon™ coated pots and pans.

Overall Health Recommendations

Enjoy twenty to forty minutes of direct sunshine every day on as much of your body as possible when available. Initially start with twenty minutes per day and incrementally go up 5 minutes every day. This is the sensible way to allow your skin to acclimate to the sun exposure over time and it will help prevent serious burns. Read the eye-opening article entitled, *Reduce your Risk of Cancer with Sunlight Exposure* by William Grant, located in the Research Archive section of this book! If you use sun-block, ONLY use organic products or simply cover yourself with light clothing to avoid burning. Conventional sunscreens and tanning lotions are believed by many statistical experts to be the number one cause of skin cancer! The toxic chemicals from them get absorbed in the body. Remember, the sun is healthy for you and is essential to combat cancer.

Fast periodically! Fasting is ABSOLUTELY ESSENTIAL in order for true detoxification to properly occur in the human body as this process efficiently facilitates the removal of waste material! Fasting can be done while supported (juice) or with just distilled water. Fasting is nature's way of cleaning up or cleansing the inside. If you reference any ancient book (Bible, Koran, etc.) they all speak of fasting in order to achieve mental and spiritual clarity along with restoring health. A couple of the best books I've read that provide instructions with a long list of scientifically validated health benefits are, *Fasting can Save your Life* by Herbert Shelton and *The Miracle of Fasting* by Paul C. Bragg. For specific, individually tailored and supported fasting program recommendations, contact me via email at **dr.matthew.loop@gmail.com**

Refrain from using tobacco products. For information on their specific harmful effects, fraudulent marketing, deceptive business practices and public relations campaigns, check out www.thetruth.com. Tobacco industry giants have been found guilty of conspiring and willingly concealing information from the public that tobacco products were known to cause cancer more than fifty years ago. These corporate giants have committed crimes against humanity by consciously choosing to sacrifice human lives for continued profits.

Breathe the purest air possible while flooding your body with oxygen. For some people this may mean getting out of clustered urban areas periodically and for many people moving. Focus on deep, belly breathing to expand the lungs to the full capacity. When we are under physical, chemical, or emotional stress, the body's natural reflex is to breathe very shallowly through our chest. This deprives the body of the proper quantities of oxygen needed to maintain a healthy internal environment. Begin to recognize this throughout the day and instead breathe deep to allow the lower portion of the ribcage and lungs to further enlarge. I recommend performing deep breathing exercises three to five times per day for at least five minutes. This will help *oxygenate* and *alkalinize* the body. Nobel Prize-winning author Dr. Otto Walberg discovered that cancer and all viruses are unable to live in an oxygen-rich environment! When your body pH is acidic, there is very little oxygen in your blood and tissues. When you flood your body with oxygen, your body pH goes from acidic to alkaline.

Meditate or pray for thirty minutes or more each day. Make a consistent effort to perform these activities intermittently throughout the day and before meals. This will put your body in a state of relaxation while allowing you to properly digest and assimilate food. Meditation also provides a powerful avenue to experience what our five senses cannot! Stress reduction will be the natural by-product of engaging in daily prayer and meditation!

Abstain from using drugs (legal or illegal)! *The use of prescription drugs, non-prescription drugs, and vaccines represent an assault on the immune system.* If you are currently taking drugs, consult your physician before you stop. Drugs of all kinds will throw off the efficient function of the GI tract. One of the most common and worse offenders are antibiotics, which disrupt the normal intestinal bacteria setting the stage for a multitude of disease producing bacteria to implant themselves. Corticosteroids are another common and terrible offender, which thin the intestinal membrane and predispose the body to the formation of ulcers and a leaky gut. Birth control and Hormone Replacement Therapy (HRT) drugs are cited in the literature as having a strong correlation in the development of cancers of the reproductive organs and breast. All drugs are toxic, foreign substances to the body and will hinder the body's ability to heal itself. In my expert opinion, drugs should only be taken in the most severe cases.

Significantly reduce or avoid exposure to Electromagnetic pollution as discussed earlier. EB 305 Cellular Cleanse therapy can assist the body in balancing & restoring its pH and electromagnetic energy. It also facilitates and aides in the detoxification process of heavy metal contaminants we are often exposed to. For more information, you can visit www.4ebr.com. Needless to say, I've seen profound results with this therapy in my office. Dr. Knox Grandison, a practitioner in the West Indies, has expanded this cutting-edge approach to detoxification and wellness throughout the Caribbean with www.dtoxcenter.com.

Exercise for at least forty-five minutes per day. Do not push yourself to exhaustion. Good health requires more than just working out in a gym, though.

Laugh and spend time with friends and family uplifting, complimenting, and giving thanks for each other.

Obtain 8 or more hours off sleep each night (very important). Healing and detoxification occur primarily at night. Go to bed before 10:00PM. We are not nocturnal beings and the more sleep you get before midnight, the more rested you'll feel the next day.

Remove yourself from *unnecessary* stressful situations. For some of this may mean switching occupations if the current one you have is unsuitable for you. If you are sick and hate your work, seriously consider doing something else, even if you are making a good wage. Your health is most important!!

- Make no excuses!
- Accept self-responsibility for your actions as well as your thoughts!

Supplement Recommendations

It is obviously best to obtain nutrients from the diet whenever possible. In my expert opinion though, nutrient supplementation is extremely important and vitally necessary in order to optimize health at a cellular level. The nutrient requirements vary from individual to individual, and are most dependent on life-style factors, genetic make-up, or health conditions.

Let me begin by saying that all supplements are *not* created equal! I continuously point this out because many individuals assume that supplements frequently purchased through grocery stores, health food markets, multi-level marketing companies, online venders, and supplement shops are all the same. This comes from a *lack of understanding* about the internal biochemistry of the human body. Our bodies are extremely intelligent when it comes to differentiating synthetic (man-made) products from the true whole food, organic form as is found in nature. You are merely paying for expensive, toxic urine when these "low-grade" products are ingested! Haphazardly consuming low quality, synthetic, preservative and dye filled, non-organic supplements will actually harm your body!

How many people actually know the difference and significance between D-ALPHA-Tocopherol and DL-ALPHA-Tocopherol? *If you are one of those that are unaware*, your health is being compromised, hence allowing another big industry to do your thinking for you! Keep in mind that the nutritional supplement industry is also a billion-dollar industry so public health is again sacrificed for profit! I use and recommend *only* 'physician-grade' products. These *superior quality* supplements can only be purchased through licensed healthcare professionals. This is the best way to ensure the quality, standardization, and *the best absorption capacity*.

If you are interested in the newest research in health and nutrition, I suggest subscribing to my FREE, monthly newsletter! All you have to do is register on my nutritional website and you will have access to my extensive research archive and my contact information via email and phone number. I'm *always available* via email to answer any questions or provide you with specific supplement recommendations based on your extensive, individual case history. These proven protocols to strengthen the immune system *must* be individually tailored for maximum results since everyone has different biochemical needs.

My nutritional website can be found at **www.matthewloop.meta-ehealth.com**

In my expert opinion, these supplements are the most important based on the traditional American lifestyle we have.

EPA/DHA (Omega 3 fish oils)—These are found in salmon, mackerel, sardines, trout, walnuts, and olives. Since the contamination of our natural resources by oils spills and other industrial wastes, I rarely recommend consuming fish anymore, but it is essential to have these fats in the diet because they play many important roles in:

- Brain development
- Energy production
- Oxygen transfer
- Prostaglandin synthesis
- Hemoglobin production
- Skin integrity and softness

They must be put through a process known as *molecular distillation* to filter out any possible contaminants. Ninety-five percent of omega 3 supplements do not undergo this process so you may wind up with an increased concentration of toxic metals if you choose to forego physician-grade quality.

Probiotics—These friendly bacteria inhabit the gut and are not traditionally found in the American diet because everything is pasteurized. Pasteurization destroys all bacteria, good or bad! Lactobacillus and Bifidobacterium are two of the more common strains that are essential for proper digestion, a strong immune system, gut motility, clotting, manufacturing B vitamins plus vitamins A and K! Fructo-oligosaccharides (FOS) should be included within a good probiotic since they provide food for our friendly microorganisms. Some common foods containing FOS include onions, chicory, garlic, leeks, asparagus, and Jerusalem artichoke.

Enzymes—Enzymes provide support in breaking down food and assimilating it into the body where it can be used to nourish the cells. Most of the food that is consumed here in our society is processed and devoid of enzymes, which is one of the main reasons why over eighty percent of Americans have digestive problems. Overeating significantly contributes as well. Furthermore, enzymes affect and greatly benefit gut motility and can go along way in preventing constipation. There is a plethora of over the counter products for the relief of digestive distress, many of which make the problems worse in the long run. It is SAFER and WISER to utilize natural digestive enzymes, which help to promote health as opposed to mere suppression of symptoms.

Chlorella—Chlorella is a single cell algae plant coming from fresh water. It is considered a super-food and a whole-food, unlike most commercial vitamins. Chlorella can help your body:

- Remove the heavy metals and other pesticides in your body
- Improve your digestive system
- Focus more clearly and for greater duration
- Balance your body's pH
- Help eliminate bad breath

As a whole-food, chlorella provides the body with an astonishing amount of nutrients that are naturally balanced and won't accumulate in your body and become toxic. This is another reason chlorella is superior to any man-made vitamin supplement

Vitamin E—Vitamin E is a premier antioxidant that:

- Decreases inflammation
- Protects cell membranes
- Assists in preventing cancer and heart disease
- Defends fatty acids from oxidative damage
- Helps with nerve and muscle function

A full spectrum vitamin E complex that contains mixed tocopherols and tocotrienols is best in terms of biological activity. I recommend avoiding supplements that list "dl-alpha-tocopherol" because it is the synthetic form of vitamin E and is greatly inferior to the natural form.

Vitamin D—Vitamin D deficiencies are common in the U.S. because many individuals do not obtain sufficient sunlight exposure to maintain adequate levels. Vitamin D functions to:

- Maintain normal blood levels of calcium and phosphorus.
- Advance bone mineralization together with other hormones, vitamins, and minerals.
- Assist in the absorption of calcium, helping to form and maintain strong bones.

Strong evidence has surfaced about the major role that Vitamin D plays in the prevention of cancer. The mechanisms by which vitamin D reduces the risk of cancer are fairly well understood. Vitamin D induces cell differentiation, increases cancer cell apoptosis or death, reduces metastasis and proliferation, and reduces angiogenesis. See *Reduce your Risk of Cancer with Sunlight Exposure* by William Grant, PhD in the research archive section of this work.

For cancer patients, the following two supplements are especially important because the human body cannot manufacture them and the standard American diet cannot provide them in sufficient amounts.

Vitamin C—Vitamin C is another leading antioxidant that:

- Stimulates the production of connective tissue throughout the body and is absolutely vital for its optimal structure.
- Assures optimal manufacturing of collagen and elastin fibers, and contributes to having tough, stable connective tissue in the human body.

A deficiency in vitamin C leads to connective tissue weakness and eventually scurvy. Experts believe that connective tissue strength has a direct relationship to the spread of cancer. The stronger the body's connective tissue, the less cancer will spread.

Lysine—an essential amino acid that:

- Stops the destruction of connective tissue by inhibiting enzymatic digestion of collagen molecules.

- Is a component of collagen and is used for collagen production in the human body.

Cancer cells secret enzymes (biocatalysts) which primarily function to digest the surrounding connective tissue at a rapid rate. This eating through the collagen fibers allows cancer to spread to different areas of the body and move freely throughout the connective tissue. *Two factors always precipitate the development of cancer.* First, the cancer cell must divide to form a growth (tumor). Secondly, enough enzymes must be produced in order to eat through the surrounding connective tissue, which allows the proliferation of the cancer. If *lysine* is absorbed in sufficient quantities, it is capable of neutralizing the destruction of the enzymes which break down the surrounding connective tissue. This occurs because lysine binds itself to the biocatalysts, similar to a lock and key mechanism, and prevents them from digesting more tissue. This may dramatically alter the progression of the disease.

Matthias Rath, MD has been the premier researcher in the field of cellular medicine. Based on scientific breakthroughs in the areas of vitamin research and cellular health, it is a direct possibility that cancer and other common diseases will be largely unknown in future generations. I encourage you to support the Dr. Rath Research Foundation's goal of establishing a new global healthcare system. (www.dr-rath-foundation.org)

PART II

8

EVERYTHING IN THE UNIVERSE IS ENERGY

E=MC²

—Albert Einstein

We are much more than what we appear to be on the surface, as modern quantum physics validates on a daily basis. *Everything* that is interpreted with the physical senses *is energy* in the form of vibration! This is one of the seven essential laws of the universe that you must be acquainted with in order to fully comprehend the magnitude and infinite nature of yourself. When we look around us, even at our own bodies, what we see is the tip of a colossal iceberg. *Everything is energy*, from a scientific perspective! Everything from the body we inhabit, the home we live in, and the money we spend is energy. In fact, everything you desire, including optimal health in abundance, is energy!

Contrary to popular belief, this is not a new concept at all. Albert Einstein, theoretical physicist widely regarded as the most important scientist of the twenty-first century, wrote the equation E=MC² in 1925.[1] One side of the equation is mass, light, and everything that we perceive with our physical senses of sight, touch, taste, smell, and hearing. All of this equals *energy*! This particular concept was, and still is profound. Quantum physics research continues to explore and apply this idea to the human body. Experts have acknowledged that there is enough energy in 1 atom of the human body to spread light throughout an entire city! At this time, let's take this a step further. I encourage you to look down at your arm for a second. Now, I know it has the tendency to appear structurally solid, but it's really not! If put under an atomic resolution microscope, you would be able to visualize the mass that is your arm vibrating at a very high frequency! The implications for this are startling!

Everything from the stars, the human body, and the car you drive is simply energy. Part of the illusion that we're living in is that we feel everything is solid when that couldn't be farther from the truth! Many things feel solid due to the rate at which the molecules are vibrating. Everything in the universe vibrates, similarly everything in the universe moves! I've heard it said many times that we are in an ocean of motion, vibratory beings in a vibratory universe so to speak.

Everything we observe with our physical senses is vibrational interpretation! In other words, you hear because your ears transmit and translate vibration. You see because your eyes translate vibration. You smell because your nose translates vibration. Our ability to touch and taste also function in accordance with vibrational interpretation. This is what enables you to perceive your environment in the way that you do! For many, this can be an extremely difficult concept to grasp, that our physical senses are not telling us the whole story. We have been taught from infancy to believe our senses but you've now been enlightened otherwise and a new secret has just been revealed!

Philosopher James Arthur Ray has stated, "If we only judged by our special senses (eyes) then we'd believe that the sun took a bath in the ocean every night, burrowed through the earth, and was reborn on the eastern shore the next morning. The ancients used to believe that! Now we know better, though. If we judged only by our sensory factors (eyes) then we would believe that the train tracks met in the distance. Again, we know better so we turn away from our senses in that example. If we only judged by our senses (ears) then we would believe a dog whistle made no sound. However, the dog comes running over after the whistle is blown." As what was just stated resonates with you, my intent is for this to begin opening your eyes a bit further. From there, the choice will be yours to find how far down the rabbit-hole leads. Too many times, when we're not careful, we find ourselves living at nothing more than the sensory level of perception.

All energy emits vibration which consequently creates a frequency! According to quantum physicists, we are frequency generators. If you get close to a persons skin, you will be able to feel infared energy given off. If you fix your eyes on them you are able to see light energy given off. Technological advances have given us different types of brain scans to actually measure the amount of energy and frequency give off. Incidentally:

- The most powerful form of all energy is THOUGHT!
- THOUGHT has the ability to penetrate all space and time.
- EVERY THOUGHT HAS A FREQUENCY!

We can actually calibrate a thought! It has been scientifically proven that thoughts have biochemical and biological properties, which means, they generate a frequency. If you're thinking that particular thought over and over again or imagining it in your mind (having abundant and vibrant health), you emit that frequency on a consistent basis.[2] If you imagine what those thoughts look and feel like, you are also emanating that frequency on a regular basis!

"Dis-ease" cannot live in a body that is alkaline and furthermore in a healthy emotional state! Cancer is no exception. If you focus and speak about your disease then ultimately you will create more cells that are in this state of dis-ease, hence you will *resonate at a low (negative) frequency.* This state of mind is completely out of balance with your natural harmony and must be identified and removed! Application of the secrets I've outlined in Chapter VIII will allow you to get in harmony, *resonate at a higher (positive) frequency,* thus permitting you to attract the vibrant health you are seeking! It is essential that we hold on to those thoughts that we *absolutely* want, while making it *perfectly* clear in our minds what we want (optimal health and healing). From that, we start to set in motion one of the greatest laws in the universe. This is THE LAW OF ATTRACTION!

9

THE UNIVERSAL LAW OF ATTRACTION

"All that we are is the result of what we have thought. The mind is everything. What we think, we become."
—**Maharishi Mahesh Yogi**

Everything that is coming into your life, you are attracting into your life whether it's good or bad! Right now that may be a bitter pill to swallow, but I assure you it's true. It's attracted to you by virtue of the images held in your mind. Your current thinking patterns regarding your abilities, how you perceive yourself, and how you live life are habitual. Many psychologists have referred to this as programming. This programming is tucked away within your subconscious mind and it dictates your behavior on a daily basis. These programs, or paradigms, came from outside sources and we often accept them without question. Frequently, our paradigm is filled with lack and limitation because a parent, instructor, coach, or another person we respected sought to protect us from disappointment. They may have conveyed words like "be realistic," "don't expect too much," "life is hard," and many other disempowering beliefs. The moment you accept their skewed lines of thinking, they start to drive your behavior and consequently limit your ability to attract abundance and prosperity in all areas of life. Plain and simply:

- YOU ATTRACT WHAT YOU'RE THINKING AND FEELING!

What we think about is ultimately what we bring about. Wise people as far back as ancient Egypt have always been aware of this universal law. It's important to assume responsibility for our conscious and subconscious thoughts while monitoring them on a daily basis! Mainstream television, radio, and newspapers are the first forms of media to start avoiding due to the negative images, fear-mongering stories, and dialogue that is continuously propagated our way. This type of media does not encourage independent, positive thinking that is needed to envision, feel, and ultimately attain vibrant health.

Like attracts like, specifically when we are referring to thought. You become and attract what you *think* and *feel* most often, like a magnet. Thoughts send out magnetic signals that are continuously drawing a parallel back to you. The most amazing feature concerning the law of attraction is, at any time, you can begin to think and create a feeling happiness and harmony. The law of attraction, in turn, will respond by drawing more things into your life that generate those positive emotions you've chosen to feel!

WHAT WE THINK ABOUT, WE BRING ABOUT

Thoughts can unquestionably heal, but they can also cause sickness and disease. Stress, which could be defined as negative thoughts, causes the internal environment of the human body to become acidic, thus setting the stage for illness and disease. These negative thoughts may manifest as conscious or unconscious in origin. Several negative thoughts are trapped in stressful or traumatic incidences from our past.

The stress of living in today's environment is higher than at any time in history. Driving a car, for example, raises stress levels in the body up to 1,000 times normal levels. When a person is driving in a car combined with talking on a cell phone, stress levels can go as high as 5,000 times the norm. Walking, conversely, actually reduces stress. Worrying about money, arguing with relatives, friends and co-workers, watching scary gruesome movies and television shows, reading the news, all increase stress levels dramatically. The good new is that it can be reversed.[1]

Visualize and feel yourself living stress-free, in abundance with vibrant health on a regular basis and you *will* attract it! Do not spend time and thoughts focusing on or speaking about disease (cancer or any other). It's no coincidence that people who tend to speak most of their illnesses or problems manifest more of the same! What differentiates the cancer survivors from those who succumb to the disease is not only positive thinking, but also consistent *visualization*. These individuals think and visualize from the end and *know* they have been cured of cancer, even before the healing may have physically manifested yet! They regularly visualize themselves in pristine health, doing the things they love, and enjoying friends and family. Visualization is the key to extraordinary health for two significant reasons: The human mind thinks in images and pictures; The unconscious mind drives your behavior. Your unconscious mind cannot differentiate between something that is real and something vividly imagined. Whatever picture you constantly think about will propel your actions to generate that exact picture. Additionally, what it comes down to is:

Happier thoughts produce a healthier biochemistry in the human body.

The groundbreaking work of pioneer researcher Dr. Masaru Emoto verifies the above concept magnificently. What has put Dr. Emoto at the forefront of the study of water is his proof that *thoughts and feelings affect physical reality*. By producing different *focused intentions* through written and spoken words and music and literally presenting it to the same water samples, the water appears to *change its expression*. Essentially, Dr. Emoto captured water's expressions. He developed a technique using a very powerful microscope in a very cold room along with high-speed photography to take pictures of newly formed crystals of frozen water samples. Not all water samples crystallize however. Water samples from extremely polluted rivers directly seem to express the state the water is in.[2]

Dr. Masaru Emoto discovered that crystals formed in frozen water reveal changes when specific, *concentrated thoughts* are directed toward them. He found that water from clear springs and water that has been exposed to loving words shows brilliant, complex, and colorful snowflake patterns. In contrast, polluted water, or water exposed to negative thoughts, forms incomplete, asymmetrical patterns with dull colors.[3] The implications of this research create a new awareness of how we can positively impact the earth and our personal health. Now, consider the fact that humans are composed of around 70 percent water! From Dr. Emoto's work and other extensive research, it becomes very clear that our thoughts, attitudes, and emotions unquestionably have an enormous effect on our body's internal environment. Negative thoughts and stress *degrade* the body and the function of our brain, which directly produces an unhealthy, acidic internal environment where illness is able to thrive. I've heard quantum physicist, Dr. John Hagelin speak in-depth on this subject numerous times.

We live in a universe based on laws and order! For example, the natural laws of the universe are so precise that NASA has no difficulty constructing spacecrafts, dispatching astronauts to the moon, and then timing the landing with the accuracy of a fraction of a second!⁴ There are no accidents or coincidence in this orderly universe. Coincidence is simply defined as that which fits together perfectly! As your mindset changes and your ability to harness abundance progresses, you will begin to realize that coincidence is nothing more than attractor energy working in your favor. You make the conscious and subconscious choice every day to attract or push away wealth in all areas of your life!

Even if you are unable comprehend the magnitude of what is being stated in this chapter, you shouldn't automatically discard it! Allow me to use electricity as a quick illustration. Do you have an understanding about how electricity works or what it really is? Even though you may not understand electricity I'm sure you enjoy and can appreciate the benefits of having it. My point is that *understanding the universal law of attraction* is the key to regaining your health from within! Once more, this is what separates the patients who miraculously go into remission and ultimately recover, from the ones that lose their struggle with cancer! The law of attraction is always working regardless if you believe or understand it. The law of attraction is THE SECRET TO VIBRANT HEALTH.

10

THE SECRET TO ATTRACTING VIBRANT HEALTH

You create your own Universe as you go along
—Winston Churchill

Below, I've listed the secrets to transforming health from the inside out. Implementing these principles will allow you to become better aligned with the universal spirit, hence permitting you to become a magnet for attracting vibrant health!

- Move away from wishing, hoping, praying, and begging for your cancer to be cured. **Know that this is a universe that works on energy and attraction!** Remind yourself that you have the power to attract the abundant health you desire. Instead use the word *intend*. Use this word when you are writing, speaking, and visualizing the following statements! Dr. Wayne Dyer, who wrote, *The Power of Intention*, elaborates in great detail, about using intention to help co-create your life as it was originally intended. I cannot recommend his book enough!

- KNOW that there is *no such thing as incurable* regardless of what stage of cancer you may be in!

- Follow the proper tenets of Nutrition as outlined in earlier chapters. This will help put your body in an alkaline environment where disease cannot thrive.

- LOVE YOURSELF profoundly! Tell yourself, "I love me" in the mirror every day! Make lists of all the wonderful things about you and add to it regularly.[1]

- THINK FROM THE END! See yourself as completely *healed* in your mind while *visualizing* yourself doing things in a complete state of perfect health. This "acting as if" will help reprogram your subconscious mind to one that attracts only vibrant health and abundance.

- Make your HAPPINESS the number one priority in your life. Happiness is a choice, not an end!

- Free yourself of any past resentments or disappointments you may be holding about you.

- LET GO of any and all resentments from the past you may be holding of everyone and everything. That which offends you only weakens you!

- NEVER talk about your illness or disease with others.

- BE GRATEFUL for the abundant health and healing that is headed your way.

- LOVE and appreciate everything and everyone, and especially yourself.

- BE CERTAIN you have the power within you to heal yourself.

- NEVER CRITICIZE OR BLAME yourself or anyone else for anything. "You cannot remedy anything by condemning it," Dr. Wayne Dyer has often stated.

- Visualize yourself as ONLY well. Perform this activity multiple times a day.

- BE HAPPY, knowing that in your state of happiness your body is healing itself.

- As you appreciate, as you love, as you are happy, as you are grateful, you are summoning well-being and it is pouring through your body and disease is vanishing in the moment.

- LAUGH! View funny movies, pictures, or recall any memories that make you laugh. Laugh your way back to health.

- MAKE LISTS every day of all the things you are grateful for, including being grateful for your healing and complete well-being.

- Do whatever you can to *remove your attention from disease.*

- Distract yourself from thoughts of disease, and *put all of your focus and attention on doing things that make you feel good.*

- LOVE EVERYHTING! Do not resist anything.

- As you love completely and feel the joy within you, disease cannot exist.
- KNOW and accept that you are PERFECT as you are right now.

In conclusion, I've made it a point to illustrate that prosperity and abundance, in the form of health, irrefutably manifests from the inside out. It is imperative that we take self-responsibility for the physical, chemical, and emotional toxins we allow into our systems on a regular basis. I stress the fact that you ultimately have the ability to free yourself from any hereditary patterns and social beliefs concerning cancer. By realizing once and for all that the power within you is greater than the power held by the world, disease will become a distant memory. In addition, we must continue to be inquisitive and seek enlightenment in all aspects of our lives! If we do not transcend our ego's definition of what we are and better understand ourselves, private interests will continue to do so and consequently health will continue to suffer. Remember, corporate giants are concerned with increased stock-prices, not public health. Keeping you sick and powerless is what facilitates this multi-billion dollar health cartel.

Make the choice to *feel good* while continuing to *empower yourself!*

APPENDIX A

CUTTING-EDGE CANCER CLINICS & RESOURCES

"All Power is from within and is therefore under our own control"
—Robert Collier

www.gerson.org (The Gerson Institute is dedicated to healing and preventing chronic and degenerative diseases based on the vision, philosophy and successful work of Max Gerson, MD. The Gerson Therapy is a powerful, natural treatment that activates the body's own healing mechanism through consuming organic vegetarian foods and juices, detoxification and natural supplements.)
Phone # 888-4-GERSON

www.cancercontrolsociety.com (Information on alternative therapies, nutrition for cancer and physician directory.)
Phone # 323-663-7801

www.oasisofhope.com (Oasis of Hope Hospital was created with the specific purpose of providing alternative cancer treatment using a multi disciplinary approach that meets the physical, emotional, and spiritual needs of the patient.)
Phone # 888-500-HOPE

www.biocarehospital.com (Integrative healthcare center of the 21st century)
Phone # 800-785-0490

www.sanoviv.com (Sanoviv is a breathtakingly beautiful, licensed medical hospital and health retreat that strives to eliminate toxins that inhibit the body's ability to heal. The Sanoviv medical team is a highly experienced, internationally trained group of physicians, nutritionists, psychologists, and fitness experts committed to treating your whole being: mind, body and soul.)

Phone # 800-726-6848

Appendix B

Recommended Readings, DVD's and Websites

1. *Cellular Health Series—Cancer:*—Matthias Rath

2. *The Cancer Industry*—Ralph Moss (http://www.ralphmoss.com/)

3. *Fats that Heal, Fats that Kill*—Udo Erasmus (http://www.fatsthatheal.com/)

4. *Dr. Mercola's Total Health Program*—Joseph Mercola (http://www.mercola.com/)

5. *Prescription for Disaster (DVD)*—Gary Null (*Prescription for Disaster* is an in-depth investigation into the symbiotic relationships between the pharmaceutical industry, the FDA, lobbyists, lawmakers, medical schools, and researchers, and the impact this has on consumers and their health care.)

6. *The Power of Intention*—Wayne Dyer (http://www.drwaynedyer.com/)

7. *Rockefeller Medicine Men*—E. Richard Brown (social-historical approach to medicine)

8. *The Safe Shopper's Bible*—David Steinman and Samuel Epstein

9. *Energy Medicine: The Scientific Basis of Bioenergy Therapies*—Candice Pert

10. *Vibrational Medicine*—Richard Gerber

11. *Natural Cures "They" Don't Want you to Know About*—Kevin Trudeau

12. *More Natural Cures Revealed*—Kevin Trudeau

13. *Digestive Wellness*—Elizabeth Lipski, (http://www.lizlipski.com/)

14. *The Food Revolution*—John Robbins (http://www.foodrevolution.org/)

15. *Lick the Sugar Habit*—Nancy Appleton (http://nancyappleton.com/)

16. *Nutrition and Physical Degeneration*—Weston A. Price (http://www.westonaprice.org/index.html)

17. *Fight for Your Health: Exposing the FDA's Betrayal of America*—Byron J. Richards

18. *Food Politics*—Marion Nestle (http://www.foodpolitics.com/)

19. *Trust Us We're Experts*—Sheldon Rampton and John Stauber

20. *Hygienic Heights*—Paul A. Goldberg (http://www.goldbergclinic.com/)

21. *Restoring Your Digestive Health*—Jordan S. Rubin

22. *Excitotoxins: The Taste that Kills*—Russell L. Blaylock

23. *Milk A-Z*—Robert Cohen

24. *Power vs. Force*—David Hawkins

25. *Fast Food Nation*—Eric Schlosser

26. *Genetically Engineered Food*—Ronnie Cummins & Ben Lilliston

27. *Dining in the Raw*—Rita Romano

28. *Mad Cowboy*—Howard Lyman (http://www.madcowboy.com/)

29. *Health Hazards of Electromagnetic Radiation*—Bruce Fife

30. *Public Exposure: DNA, Democracy, and the Wireless Revolution (DVD)*—directed by James Heddle (*Public Exposure* is a dramatic video report on cell phone and cell tower microwave technology now proliferating internationally, its sobering potential effects on human health and democracy, and what citizens and responsible officials around the world are doing to respond.)

31. *Electromagnetic Fields*—B. Blake Levitt

32. *Healing with Magnets*—Gary Null

33. *Flood your Body with Oxygen*—Ed McCabe (http://www.oxygenhealth.com/)

34. *The Drug Story*—Morris A. Bealle

35. *Walden*—Henry D. Thoreau

36. *Water can Undermine Your Health*—Norman Walker

37. *The Medical Mafia*—Guylaine Lanctot

38. *Quantum Touch: The Power to Heal*—Richard Gordon

39. *Energy Medicine*—James L. Oschman

40. *Living in the Raw*—Rose Lee Calabro

41. *The History of a Crime Against the Food Law*—Harvey W. Wiley

42. *Racketeering in Medicine: The Suppression of Alternatives*—James P. Carter

43. *It's All in Your Head: The link between Mercury Amalgams and Illness*—Hal. A. Huggins

44. *Fluoride: The Aging Factor*—John Yiamouyannis

45. *The Joy of Juicing*—Gary Null

46. *The Crime and Punishment of I.G. Farben*—Joseph Borkin

47. *1001 All-Natural Secrets to a Pest-Free Property*—Myles H. Bader (natural pest control)

48. *Cancer Doesn't Scare me Anymore*—Lorriane Day (www.drday.com/ (A former San Francisco surgeon who beat cancer through diet and an unshakable belief in God and Spirit to heal those who wish to be healed.)

49. *Sweet Misery: A Poisoned World (DVD)*—a film by Cori Brackett (A compelling documentary that exposes the real dangers of Aspartame and how it became FDA approved.)

Helpful Websites

www.matthewloop.meta-ehealth.com (Register on my secure, exclusive website and I will send you FREE monthly newsletters, via email, so you can stay abreast of the newest, cutting-edge information concerning nutrition, medicine and alternative medicine research, as well as fitness.)

www.dtoxcenter.com (The DtoxCenter was created to help individuals achieve optimal health and well being by administration of the detoxifying "Energy Balancer" cellular cleanse foot bath.)

www.wholefoodsmarket.com (The world's leading retailer of natural and organic foods.)

www.mercola.com (Free weekly newsletter of top medical news on subjects including cause, prevention and alternative treatment for a variety of common medical conditions.)

www.educate-yourself.org (website for *The Freedom of Knowledge and The Power of Thought*)

www.garynull.com (Gary Null PhD empowers all who will listen with life-changing information that promote heath and wellness)

www.dr-rath-foundation.org (The leading resource of natural health information for patients, health professionals and health politicians everywhere.)

www.whatthebleep.com

www.thecorporation.com

www.naturalcures.com (The Natural Cures[TM] website provides you with information about non-drug, non-surgical and all-natural cures that drug companies and government agencies DO NOT want you to know about.)

www.redflagsdaily.com/index.php

www.drwaynedyer.com

www.price-pottenger.org

www.thetruth.com

www.truthaboutsplenda.com

www.supersizeme.com

www.rawfood.com

www.organicconsumers.org/

www.iaomt.org (International Academy of Oral Medicine and Toxicology promotes mercury-free and biological dentistry—directory by state included)

www.rife.org

www.jamesray.com (create wealth in all areas of your life)

APPENDIX C

VIBRANT HEALTH NUTRITIONAL & LIFESTYLE REFERENCE

I have included some very valuable resources in this section that will enable you to take back your health and drastically reduce the *total toxic load* on your body. This will empower you and allow you to make good food choices based on the few superior quality products that are available to us. Whole Foods Market, Wild Oats Market, and many smaller organic grocers carry many of these food, body, and home-care products in their stores. Online and phone-in ordering is available for most of these products.

Food and Beverage Products

Red Meat

Eat Wild
Explains the benefits of eating meat and dairy products from grass-fed, not grain-fed animals. On their suppliers' page, you can find out how to purchase grass-fed meat and dairy products in your area
www.eatwild.com

White Egret Farm
Offers unprocessed natural beef, goat, and free-range turkeys, as well as goat dairy products.
-    Telephone: (512) 276.7408 or (512) 276-7505
www.whiteegretfarm.com

Coleman Natural Meats
Naturally raised, hormone and antibiotic free beef products.

- Telephone: (800) 442.8666

www.colemannatural.com

Brady Axis Venison

Pasture-fed venison
- Telephone: (800) 291.9555

www.ehunter.com/brady

Organic Valley

Packaged organic steaks and hot dogs
- Telephone: (608) 625.2602

www.organicvalley.com

Maverick Ranch Natural Meats

Natural beef, chicken, lamb, and buffalo
- Telephone: (303) 294.0146

www.maverickranch.com

Poultry

Applegate Farms

Packaged chicken and turkey deli slices
- Telephone: (800) 587.8289

www.applegatefarms.com

Bell & Evans

Fresh and frozen poultry products
- Telephone: (717) 865.1176

www.bellandevans.com

White Egret Farm

Offers unprocessed natural beef, goat, and free-range turkeys, as well as goat dairy products.
- Telephone: (512) 276.7408 or (512) 276-7505

www.whiteegretfarm.com

Oaklyn Plantation

Offers free-range chicken raised without antibiotics or growth hormones

- Telephone: (843) 395.0793
www.freerangechicken.com

Shelton's Poultry
   Turkey and chicken, free-range, antibiotic and hormone free
   - Telephone: (909) 623.4361
www.sheltons.com

Dairy Products

White Egret Farm
   Offers raw hard and soft goat cheeses and Probiogurt, a 30 hour raw goats milk yogurt containing beneficial microorganisms, enzymes, and highly digestible protein.
   - Telephone: (512) 276.7408 or (512) 276-7505
www.whiteegretfarm.com

Redwood Hill Farm
   Offers pasteurized goat's milk yogurt and cheeses.
   - Telephone: (707) 823.8250
www.redwoodhill.com

Real Foods Market
   Offers raw, organic dairy products from grass-fed cows. Products include cream, butter, yogurt, kefir, and cheeses. These products can be purchased via mail order and are shipped frozen
   - Telephone: (866) 284.7325
www.realfoodsmarket.com

Organic Pastures
   Offers organic, raw dairy products from grass-fed cows.
   - Telephone: (559) 846.9732
www.organicpastures.com

Natural By Nature
   Offers grass-fed, organic cream, soft cheeses, cream cheese, sour cream, and butter.

- Telephone: (610) 268.6962

www.natural-by-nature.com

Helios Nutrition
   Certified organic plain low-fat kefir.
   - Telephone: (651) 436.2914

www.heliosnutrition.com

Stonyfield Farm
   Certified organic whole-milk plain
   - Telephone: (603) 437.5050

www.stonyfield.com

Fish

Real Foods Market
   Offers wild salmon and salmon jerky available frozen by mail order.
   - Telephone: (866) 284.7325

www.realfoodsmarket.com

Barlean's Fishery
   Offers ecologically wild harvested salmon, a rich source of omega 3 fatty acids.
   - Telephone: (360) 384.0485

www.barleans.com

Crown Prince Natural
   Offers canned sardines, herring, tuna, and salmon.
   - Telephone: (626) 912-5850

www.crownprince.com

Ecofish, Inc.
   Offers ocean-caught salmon, halibut, tuna, and other fish.
   - Telephone: (603) 430.0101

www.ecofish.com

Eggs

Organic Valley
    Certified organic, high omega 3 eggs.
    -    Telephone: (608) 625.2602
www.organicvalley.com

Pete and Gerry's Organic Eggs
    Locally produced farm-fresh eggs from free-range chickens.
    -    Telephone: (800) 438. 3447
www.peteandgerrys.com

Gold Circle Farms
    Offers DHA, omega 3 eggs.
www.goldcirclefarms.com

Nuts and Seeds

The Almond Brothers
    -    Telephone: (207) 780.1101
www.organicglobal.com

Glaser Organic Farms
    Offers an extensive supply of organic raw nuts and seeds.
    -    Telephone: (305) 238. 7747
www.glaserorganicfarms.com

Silver Spring Supplements
    Offers an extensive supply of organic, raw nuts and seeds.
    -    Telephone: (800) 520.1791
www.silverspringsupplements.com

The Raw World
    Offers supplies of raw foods, live food supplements, juicers, blenders, and many other great products.
    -    Telephone: (866) RAW.DIET
www.therawworld.com

Nut and Seed Butters

Rejuvenative Foods
Offers high quality raw, organic, nut and seed butters, including butters made from almond, sesame, pumpkin, cashew, and sunflower seeds.
-    Telephone: (800) 805.7957
www.rejuvenative.com

Glaser Organic Farms
Offers an extensive supply of organic raw nuts and seed butters.
-    Telephone: (305) 238.7747
www.glaserorganicfarms.com

Maranatha
Offers organic nut and seed butters.
www.maranatha.com

The Raw World
Offers supplies of raw foods, live food supplements, juicers, blenders, and many other great products.
-    Telephone: (866) RAW.DIET
www.therawworld.com

Healthy Fats and Oils

Garden of Life
Offers extra-virgin Coconut Oil, an unheated, certified organic oil produced using traditional fermentation methods. This premier oil contains 52-55% lauric acid.
-    Telephone: (866) 465.0094 (for nearest retailer in your area)
www.gardenoflifeusa.com

Barlean's Organic Oils
Offers organic, high lignan flaxseed oil and barrage seed oil.
-    Telephone: (360) 384.0485
www.barleans.com

Omega Nutrition
> Offers organic flax oil, olive oil, and organic garlic-chili flax oil
> - Telephone: (800) 661.3529

www.omeganutrition.com

Flora, Inc.
> Offers organic oils in glass bottles, including hard-to-find oils.
> - Telephone: (800) 498.3610

www.florahealth.com

The Raw World
> Offers supplies of raw foods, live food supplements, juicers, blenders, and many other great products.
> - Telephone: (866) RAW.DIET

www.therawworld.com

Spectrum Naturals
> Offers organic extra-virgin olive oil.
> - Telephone: (707) 778.8900

www.spectrumorganic.com

Organic Produce (Fresh and Frozen)

Earthbound Farms
> Offers fresh, packaged organic produce
> - Telephone: (800) 690.3200

www.earthboundfarm.com

Cascadian Farms
> Offers frozen, packaged organic fruits and vegetables, including frozen, organic berries.
> - Telephone: (360) 855.2730

www.cfarm.com

Champlain Valley Farms
> Offers frozen, packaged fruits and vegetables
> - Telephone: (613) 674.2444

Seaweed

Eden Foods
- Telephone: (800) 248.0320

www.edenfoods.com

Island Herbs and Kelp
Offers fine hand-harvested bullwhip kelp and bladderwrack seaweed from moving cold water in the Pacific Northwest.
Email: ryandrum2020@yahoo.com

Maine Coast
- Telephone: (207) 565.2907

www.seaveg.com

Produce Washes

Bi-O-Kleen
- Telephone: (503) 557.0216

www.bi-o-kleen.com

Seventh Generation
- Telephone (802) 658.3773

www.seventhgeneration.com

Vegetables (in Glass Jars)

BioNaturae
Offers whole tomatoes peeled, crushed, stewed, and tomato paste in glass jars
- Telephone: (860) 642.6996

www.bionaturae.com

Mediterranean Organics
Offers organic red peppers, dehydrated organic sun-dried tomatoes in organic olive oil with spices and capers. All are packaged in glass jars.
- Telephone: (914) 232. 3102

www.mediterraneanorganic.com

Muir Glen
  Offers canned tomato products, tomato sauces, and salsas.
  -   Telephone: (800) 832.6345
www.muirglen.com

Dried Fruit

Glaser Organic Farms
  Offers organic dried fruits.
  -   Telephone: (305) 238.7747
www.glaserorganicfarms.com

Himalania
  Offers organic dried goji berries as well as unrefined Himalayan crystal salt
http://www.himalania.com

Silver Spring Supplements
  Offers organic dried fruits.
  -   Telephone: (800) 520.1791
www.silverspringsupplements.com

Woodstock Organics
  -   Telephone: (914) 623.7649
www.woodstockorganics.com

Pavich Family Farms
  -   Telephone: (661) 391.6354
www.pavich.com

Fruit Spreads/Applesauce

BioNaturae
  Offers high quality organic fruit spreads.
  -   Telephone: (860) 642.6996
www.bionaturae.com

Cascadian Farms
  Offers organic fruit spreads.

- Telephone: (360) 855.2730
www.cfarm.com

Eden Foods
Offers high quality, organic apple sauce.
- Telephone: (800) 248.0320
www.edenfoods.com

Santa Cruz Organic
Offers organic apple sauce.
- Telephone: (530) 899.5000
www.knudsenjuices.com

Salt and Seasonings

Himalania
Offers unrefined Himalayan crystal salt
http://www.himalania.com

The Grain and Salt Society
Offers Celtic Sea salt and other health food products.
- Telephone: (800) 867.7258
www.celticseasalt.com

Le Tresor
Offers certified organic sea salt
- Telephone: (415) 761.7122
www.saltworks.us

Frontier Herbs
Offers organic spices in glass jars
- Telephone: (800) 669.3275
www.frontiernaturalbrands.com

Spice Hunter
Offers packaged organic spices in glass jars.
- Telephone: (800) 444.3096
www.spicehunter.com

Rapunzel Pure Organics
Offers a good selection of seasonings made with sea salt and organic herbs.
- Telephone: (518) 392.8620
www.rapunzel.com

Sweeteners

Wisdom of the Ancients
Offers Stevia products (safe for diabetics)
- Telephone: (480) 921.1373
www.wisdomherbs.com

Shady Maple
Offers organic maple syrup.
- Telephone: (905) 206.1455
www.shadymaple.ca

Wholesome Foods
Offers sucanat organic unrefined sugar
- Telephone: (281) 490.9582
www.wholesomesweeteners.com

Rapunzel Pure Organics
Offers rapadura organic unrefined sugar.
- Telephone: (518) 392.8620
www.rapunzel.com

Honey

Really Raw Honey Company
Offers the finest enzyme-rich raw honey.
- Telephone: (800) 732.5729
www.reallyrawhoney.com

Northwoods Apiaries
Offers certified organic raw honey, pollen, propolis, and beeswax.

- Telephone: (802) 744.2007

Email: jwhite@surfglobal.net

Farm Style Raw Apitherapy Honey
Offers raw honey, propolis, and other bee products.
- Telephone: (802) 985.5852

www.honeygardens.com/contact.htm

Manuka Honey USA
Offers a variety of raw honey products.
- Telephone: (541) 902.0979

www.manukahoneyusa.com

Apple Cider and Other Vinegars

Spectrum Naturals
Offers organic balsamic, cider, brown rice, and wine vinegars.
- Telephone: (707) 778.8900

www.spectrumorganic.com

Bragg Apple Cider Vinegar
Offers apple cider vinegar made from organically grown apples, as well as other natural products.
- Telephone: (800) 446.1990

BioNaturae
Offers organic balsamic vinegar.
- Telephone: (860) 642.6996

www.bionaturae.com

Condiments

Spectrum Organic Products
Offers health organic omega 3 mayonnaise using expeller pressed soy and flax-seed oils.
- Telephone: (707) 778.8900

www.spectrumorganic.com

Roland Foods
-     Telephone: (800) 221.4030
www.rolandfood.com

Westbrae Natural Foods
Offers natural catsup and mustard.
-     Telephone: (562) 948.2872
www.novelco.com/westbrae/index.htm

Dream Foods International
Offers organic volcano lemon burst, lemon juice with lemon oil.
-     Telephone: (310) 392.6324
www.dreamfoods.com

Heinz Foods
-     Telephone: (800) 255.5750
www.heinz.com

Soups

Walnut Acres/Acirca Inc.
-     Telephone: (916) 791.7334
www.walnutacres.com

Amy's Kitchen
-     Telephone: (707) 578.7188
www.amys.com

Anke Kruse Organics
Offers Sun organic dried soups.
-     Telephone: (519) 853.3899
www.ankekruseorganics.ca

Shariann's Organic
-     Telephone: (800) 434.4246
www.shariannsorganic.com

Dried/Canned Soup Stocks

Anke Kruse Organics
>Offers harvest sun organic chicken bouillon cubes.
> -   Telephone: (519) 853.3899

www.ankekruseorganics.ca

Pacific Foods
>Offers certified organic free-range chicken stock.
> -   Telephone: (503) 692.9666

www.pacificfoods.com

Health Valley
>Offers beef and chicken stock in cans.
> -   Telephone: (516) 237.6200

www.hain-celestial.com

Marinades

Chelten House Products
>Offers organic sauces, dressings, and marinades
> -   Telephone: (856) 467.1600

www.cheltenhouse.com

Spectrum Naturals
>Offers refrigerated organic dips and spreads.
> -   Telephone: (707) 778.8900

www.spectrumorganic.com

Glaser Organic Farms
> -   Telephone: (305) 238.7747

www.glaserorganicfarms.com

Sauces

Walnut Acres/Acirca Inc.
>Offers organic salsas.

- Telephone: (916) 791.7334

www.walnutacres.com

Muir Glen
Offers organic tomato sauces and salsas.
- Telephone: (800) 832.6345

www.muirglen.com

Seeds of Change
Offers organic tomato sauces and salsas.
- Telephone: (888) 762.4240

www.seedsofchange.com

Wizard Organic Sauces
Offers organic vegetarian Worcestershire sauce and hot sauce
- Telephone: (805) 684.8500

www.edwardandsons.com

Pasta's

BioNaturae
Offers organic whole grain pasta's from Italy.
- Telephone: (860) 642.6996

www.bionaturae.com

Rizopia
Offers organic wild rice and organic corn pasta.
- Telephone: (416) 609-8820

www.rizopia.com

Eden Foods
- Telephone: (800) 248.0320

www.edenfoods.com

Eddies Pastas
- Telephone: (858) 486.1101

www.mrsleeperspasta.com

Tinkyada Pastas
    Offers wheat/gluten free.
    -    Telephone: (416) 609.0016
www.tinkyada.com

Coconut Milk

Native Forest
    Offers certified organic coconut milk.
    -    Telephone: (805) 684.8500
www.edwardandsons.com

Cereals

Kashi Company
    -    Telephone: (858) 274.8870
www.kashi.com

Foods for Life
    Offers high quality sprouted cereals, including Ezekial 4:9 cereal
    -    Telephone: (909) 279.5090
www.food-for-life.com

Natures Path
    -    Telephone: (604) 940.0505
www.naturespath.com

Save the Forest
    Offers packaged organic granolas
    -    Telephone: (800) 910.2884
www.nenb.com

Grains and Flour

Lundberg Family Farms
    Offers packaged and bulk organic grains and flour.
    -    Telephone: (530) 882.4551
www.lundberg.com

Arrowhead Mills
>   Offers packaged and bulk organic grains and flour.
>   - Telephone: (800) 749.0730
>   www.arrowheadmills.com

Breads

Foods for Life
>   Offers high quality sprouted breads (Ezekial bread), bagels, and tortillas
>   - Telephone: (909) 279.5090
>   www.food-for-life.com

Natures Path
>   Produces of manna sprouted grain bread.
>   - Telephone: (604) 940.0505
>   www.naturespath.com

French Meadow Bakery
>   Offers organic yeast free breads.
>   - Telephone: (612) 870.4740
>   www.frenchmeadow.com

Alvarado Street Bakery
>   Offers sprouted breads, tortillas, and bagels
>   - Telephone: (707) 585.3293
>   www.alvaradostbakery.com

Bottled Fruit Beverages

BioNaturae
>   Offers organic bottled juices from Italy.
>   - Telephone: (860) 642.6996
>   www.bionaturae.com

Dream Foods International
>   Offers Italian organic volcano orange juice and organic blood orange juice that's high in antioxidants.

-    Telephone: (310) 392.6324
www.dreamfoods.com

POM Wonderful
Offers pomegranate juice
-    Telephone: (310) 966.5800
www.pomwonderful.com

Austria's Finest Naturally
Offers Austrian black currant juice that's a rich source of antioxidants
-    Telephone: (703) 780.8393
www.austrianpumkinoil.com

GTS Kombucha and Synergy Drinks
Offers organic, fermented beverages.
-    Telephone: (877) RE-JUICE
www.naturezone.net

Teas

Choice Teas
Offers organic herbal teas.
-    Telephone: (800) 882.8943

Yogi Teas
Offers organic herbal teas.
-    Telephone: (800) 964.4832
www.yogitea.com

Long Life Teas
Offers organic herbal teas.
-    Telephone: (800) 645.5768
www.long-life.com

Numi Tea
Offers certified organic full leaf teas and fresh herbs
-    Telephone: (510) 567.8903
www.numitea.com

One World Teas
Offers organic Japanese teas.
-    Telephone: (828) 665.7790
www.great-eastern-sun.com

Snacks

Organic Food Bar, Inc.
Offers certified organic living food bars
-    Telephone: (800) 246.4685
www.organicfoodbar.com

Bio International
-    Telephone: (800) 246.4685
www.organicfoodbar.com

The Raw World
Offers raw food snacks.
-    Telephone: (866) RAW-DIET
www.therawworld.com

Jennie's Macaroons
Offers snack that are made with only three ingredients: coconut, honey, and egg whites with a higher amount of lauric acid.
-    Telephone: (718) 384.2150
www.redmillfarms.com

Anke Kruse Organics
Offers wild country organic honey and nut bars.
-    Telephone: (519) 853.3899
www.ankekruseorganics.ca

Organic Chocolate Spreads
-    Telephone: (800) 805.7957
www.rejuvenative.com

Non-Toxic Body-Care Products

Dental Products

Jason Naturals
-    Telephone: (877) 527.6601
www.jason-natural.com

Weleda
-    Telephone: (845) 268.8599
www.weleda.com

Eco-Dent
-    Telephone: (888) 326.3368
www.eco-dent.com

Uncle Harry's
-    Telephone: (425) 643.4664
www.uncleharrys.com

Skin and Body Products

Aubrey Organics
Aubrey Organics is the leading supplier of organic skin and body care products. Aubrey Organics is a voice for truth in the skin and body-care industry. They produce hundreds of products including skin-care, hair-care, soaps and cleansers, toothpaste, natural hair color, and much more.
-    Telephone: (813) 877.4186
www.aubrey-organics.com

Kiss My Face
Offers organic product lines and olive oil soap bars.
-    Telephone: (845) 255.0884
www.kissmyface.com

Tropical Traditions
Offers high quality skin and body care products made from virgin coconut oil and other high quality ingredients.

- Telephone: (866) 311.2626
www.tropicaltraditions.com

Weleda
Offers spray deodorants
- Telephone: (845) 268.8599
www.weleda.com

Jason Naturals
- Telephone: (877) 527.6601
www.jason-natural.com

Mychelle Dermaceuticals
Provides high quality effective skin and body care products. This company utilizes innovative fruit and vegetables and their enzymes to deliver outstanding results for men and women.
- Telephone: (800) 447.2076
www.mychelleusa.com

Dr. Bronners
Provides liquid soaps
- Telephone: (760) 743.2211

Sunscreens

Garden of Life
Offers certified organic extra-virgin coconut oil used by tropical cultures to prevent sunburn and as a key ingredient in commercial sunscreens
- Telephone: (866) 465.0094
www.gardenoflifeusa.com

Aubrey Organics
- Telephone: (813) 877.4186
www.aubrey-organics.com

Feminine Products

Life-Flo
  Offers natural care for men and women.
  -    Telephone: (602) 995.8715
www.life-flo.com

Organic Essentials
  Also produces organic cotton balls and cotton swabs
  -    Telephone: (800) 765.6491
www.organicessentials.com

Natracare
  -    Telephone: (303) 617.3476
www.natracare.com

Non-Toxic Hair Color

Aubrey Organics
  -    Telephone: (813) 877.4186
www.aubrey-organics.com

Light Mountain
  -    Telephone: (800) 548.3824
www.lotuslight.com

Bath Salts and Oils

Common Sense Farm
  Provides great bath salts.
  -    Telephone: (518) 677.0224
www.commonsensefarm.com

Dead Sea Bath Salts
  -    Telephone: (818) 717.8300
www.masada.spa.com

Home-Care Products

EMF Reducers

Cutting Edge Catalog
- Telephone: (800) 497.9516

www.cutcat.com

Real Goods Catalog
- Telephone: (800) 762.7325

Less EMF Catalog
- Telephone: (888) 537.7363

www.lessemf.com

Shower Filtration

New Wave Enviro Products
Provides shower chlorine filters and much more.
- Telephone: (800) 592.8371

www.newwaveenviro.com/Filters.html

Aquasana
- Telephone: (817) 536.5250

www.aquasana.com

Care Free Technologies
- Telephone: (714) 545.4500

www.carefreewater.com

Air Purification

Pionair Air Purifiers
Provides increased quality of air in the home and reduces harmful toxins such as yeast, molds, bacteria, and debris.
- Telephone: (866) PIONAIR

www.pionair.net

Nikken, Inc.
   Offers filter systems, including HEPA 3, which is used in operating rooms.
   -   Telephone: (949) 789.2000
www.nikken.com

Health More
   -   Telephone: (216) 432.1990
www.filterclean.com

Austin Air Systems
   Removes both gases and odors. Medical HEPA and granulated carbon filters.
   -   Telephone: (800) 724.8403
www.austinair.com

N.E.E.D.S.
   -   Telephone: (800) 634.1380
www.needs.com

Full Spectrum Lighting

Seventh Generation
   -   Telephone: (802) 658.3773
www.seventhgeneration.com

Chromalux
   -   Telephone: (800) 354.5596
www.lumiram.com

Household Products (Dish, Laundry, & Cleaning)

Seventh Generation
   -   Telephone: (802) 658.3773
www.seventhgeneration.com

Earth Friendly Products
   -   Telephone: (800) 335.3267
www.ecos.com

Heather's Oxygen Bleach
Provides a non-toxic alternative to Comet or Ajax
- Telephone: (310) 838.7543

www.jason-natural.com

TKO Orange
All purpose cleaner and stain and odor remover made only from organic orange oil.
- Telephone: (800) 995.2463

www.tkoorange.com

Sal Suds
Offers all purpose cleaners, great for laundry, dishes, and general household cleaning.
- Telephone: (760) 743.2211

Life Tree Products
- Telephone: (800) 347.5211

www.goturtle.com

Bi-O-Kleen
- Telephone: (503) 557.0216

www.bi-o-kleen.com

Flora, Inc.
Offers Turbo plus Ceramic Laundry Discs and Flora Brite papaya enzyme laundry additive and whitener.
- Telephone: (800) 498.3610

www.florahealth.com

Cookware and Household Appliances

Green Mountain Soapstone
Soapstone cookware heats very quickly and has remarkable heat retention properties, which creates a more even cooking surface. Because soapstone is non-porous, it also has a natural nonstick surface.

I also recommend stainless steel or waterless cookware.

- Telephone: (802) 468.5636

www.greenmountainsoapstone.com

Vita-Mix Blender

Offers a very high quality durable blender that is excellent for smoothies.
- Telephone: (800) 848. 2649

www.vitamix.com

Ronco Yogurt Maker and Food Dehydrator
- Telephone: (800) 486.1806

www.ronco.com

Aroma Convection Ovens

Offers multi-purpose, healthy cooking, "microwave speed," Convection Ovens and much more.
- Telephone—(858) 587-8866

www.aromaco.com/

Organic Pet Food and Treats

Only Natural Pet Store

Offers an outstanding array of quality organic products for your pet including dog and cat food, treats, holistic remedies, supplements, shampoos, and much more.
- Telephone: (888) 937.6677

www.onlynaturalpet.com

Organic Pet Products

Provides an outstanding array of quality organic products for your pet including dog and cat food, treats, holistic remedies, supplements, shampoos, and much more.

www.organicpetproducts.com

Cancer Research Archive

Cancer's Sweet Tooth

Patrick Quillin, PHD, RD, CNS

During the last 10 years I have worked with more than 500 cancer patients as director of nutrition for Cancer Treatment Centers of America in Tulsa, Okla. It puzzles me why the simple concept "sugar feeds cancer" can be so dramatically overlooked as part of a comprehensive cancer treatment plan.

Of the 4 million cancer patients being treated in America today, hardly any are offered any scientifically guided nutrition therapy beyond being told to "just eat good foods." Most patients I work with arrive with a complete lack of nutritional advice. I believe many cancer patients would have a major improvement in their outcome if they controlled the supply of cancer's preferred fuel, glucose. By slowing the cancer's growth, patients allow their immune systems and medical debulking therapies—chemotherapy, radiation and surgery to reduce the bulk of the tumor mass—to catch up to the disease. Controlling one's blood-glucose levels through diet, supplements, exercise, meditation and prescription drugs when necessary can be one of the most crucial components to a cancer recovery program. The sound bite—sugar feeds cancer—is simple. The explanation is a little more complex.

The 1931 Nobel laureate in medicine, German Otto Warburg, Ph.D., first discovered that cancer cells have a fundamentally different energy metabolism compared to healthy cells. The crux of his Nobel thesis was that malignant tumors frequently exhibit an increase in anaerobic glycolysis—a process whereby glucose is used as a fuel by cancer cells with lactic acid as an anaerobic byproduct—compared to normal tissues.[1] The large amount of lactic acid produced by this fermentation of glucose from cancer cells is then transported to the liver. This conversion of glucose to lactate generates a lower, more acidic pH in cancerous tissues as well as overall physical fatigue from lactic acid buildup.[2,3] Thus, larger tumors tend to exhibit a more acidic pH.[4]

This inefficient pathway for energy metabolism yields only 2 moles of adenosine triphosphate (ATP) energy per mole of glucose, compared to 38 moles of ATP in the complete aerobic oxidation of glucose. By extracting only about 5 percent (2 vs. 38 moles of ATP) of the available energy in the food supply and the body's calorie stores, the cancer is "wasting" energy, and the patient becomes tired and undernourished. This vicious cycle increases body wasting.[5] It is one reason why 40 percent of cancer patients die from malnutrition, or cachexia.[6]

Hence, cancer therapies should encompass regulating blood-glucose levels via diet, supplements, non-oral solutions for cachectic patients who lose their appetite, medication, exercise, gradual weight loss and stress reduction. Professional guidance and patient self-discipline are crucial at this point in the cancer process. The quest is not to eliminate sugars or carbohydrates from the diet but rather to control blood glucose within a narrow range to help starve the cancer and bolster immune function.

The glycemic index is a measure of how a given food affects blood-glucose levels, with each food assigned a numbered rating. The lower the rating, the slower the digestion and absorption process, which provides a healthier, more gradual infusion of sugars into the bloodstream. Conversely, a high rating means blood-glucose levels are increased quickly, which stimulates the pancreas to secrete insulin to drop blood-sugar levels. This rapid fluctuation of blood-sugar levels is unhealthy because of the stress it places on the body (see glycemic index chart).

Sugar in the Body and Diet

Sugar is a generic term used to identify simple carbohydrates, which includes monosaccharides such as fructose, glucose and galactose; and disaccharides such as maltose and sucrose (white table sugar). Think of these sugars as different-shaped bricks in a wall. When fructose is the primary monosaccharide brick in the wall, the glycemic index registers as healthier, since this simple sugar is slowly absorbed in the gut, then converted to glucose in the liver. This makes for "time-release foods," which offer a more gradual rise and fall in blood-glucose levels. If glucose is the primary monosaccharide brick in the wall, the glycemic index will be higher and less healthy for the individual. As the brick wall is torn apart in digestion, the glucose is pumped across the intestinal wall directly into the bloodstream, rapidly raising blood-glucose levels. In other words, there is a "window of efficacy" for glucose in the blood: levels too low make one feel lethargic and can create clinical hypoglycemia; levels too high start creating the rippling effect of diabetic health problems.

The 1997 American Diabetes Association blood-glucose standards consider 126 mg glucose/dL blood or greater to be diabetic; 111-125 mg/dL is impaired glucose tolerance and less than 110 mg/dL is considered normal. Meanwhile, the Paleolithic diet of our ancestors, which consisted of lean meats, vegetables and small amounts of whole grains, nuts, seeds and fruits, is estimated to have generated blood glucose levels between 60 and 90 mg/dL.[7] Obviously, today's high-sugar diets are having unhealthy effects as far as blood-sugar is concerned. Excess blood glucose may initiate yeast overgrowth, blood vessel deterioration, heart disease and other health conditions.[8]

Understanding and using the glycemic index is an important aspect of diet modification for cancer patients. However, there is also evidence that sugars may feed cancer more efficiently than starches (comprised of long chains of simple sugars), making the index slightly misleading. A study of rats fed diets with equal calories from sugars and starches, for example, found the animals on the high-sugar diet developed more cases of breast cancer.[9] The glycemic index is a useful tool in guiding the cancer patient toward a healthier diet, but it is not infallible. By using the glycemic index alone, one could be led to thinking a cup of white sugar is healthier than a baked potato. This is because the glycemic index rating of a sugary food may be lower than that of a starchy food. To be safe, I recommend less fruit, more vegetables, and little to no refined sugars in the diet of cancer patients.

What the Literature Says

A mouse model of human breast cancer demonstrated that tumors are sensitive to blood-glucose levels. Sixty-eight mice were injected with an aggressive strain of breast cancer, then fed diets to induce either high blood-sugar (hyperglycemia), normoglycemia or low blood-sugar (hypoglycemia). There was a dose-dependent response in which the lower the blood glucose, the greater the survival rate. After 70 days, 8 of 24 hyperglycemic mice survived compared to 16 of 24 normoglycemic and 19 of 20 hypoglycemic.[10] This suggests that regulating sugar intake is key to slowing breast tumor growth (see chart).

In a human study, 10 healthy people were assessed for fasting blood-glucose levels and the phagocytic index of neutrophils, which measures immune-cell ability to envelop and destroy invaders such as cancer. Eating 100 g carbohydrates from glucose, sucrose, honey and orange juice all significantly decreased the capacity of neutrophils to engulf bacteria. Starch did not have this effect.[11]

A four-year study at the National Institute of Public Health and Environmental Protection in the Netherlands compared 111 biliary tract cancer patients with 480 controls. Cancer risk associated with the intake of sugars, independent of other energy sources, more than doubled for the cancer patients.[12] Furthermore, an epidemiological study in 21 modern countries that keep track of morbidity and mortality (Europe, North America, Japan and others) revealed that sugar intake is a strong risk factor that contributes to higher breast cancer rates, particularly in older women.[13]

Limiting sugar consumption may not be the only line of defense. In fact, an interesting botanical extract from the avocado plant (*Persea americana*) is showing promise as a new cancer adjunct. When a purified avocado extract called manno-heptulose was added to a number of tumor cell lines tested in vitro by researchers in the Department of Biochemistry at Oxford University in Britain, they found it inhibited tumor cell glucose uptake by 25 to 75 percent, and it inhibited the enzyme glucokinase responsible for glycolysis. It also inhibited the growth rate of the cultured tumor cell lines. The same researchers gave lab animals a 1.7 mg/g body weight dose of mannoheptulose for five days; it reduced tumors by 65 to 79 percent.[14] Based on these studies, there is good reason to believe that avocado extract could help cancer patients by limiting glucose to the tumor cells.

Since cancer cells derive most of their energy from anaerobic glycolysis, Joseph Gold, M.D., director of the Syracuse (N.Y.) Cancer Research Institute and former U.S. Air Force research physician, surmised that a chemical called hydrazine sulfate, used in rocket fuel, could inhibit the excessive gluconeogenesis (making sugar from amino acids) that occurs in cachectic cancer patients. Gold's work demonstrated hydrazine sulfate's ability to slow and reverse cachexia in advanced cancer patients. A placebo-controlled trial followed 101 cancer patients taking either 6 mg hydrazine sulfate three times/day or placebo. After one month, 83 percent of hydrazine sulfate patients increased their weight, compared to 53 percent on placebo.[15] A similar study by the same principal researchers, partly funded by the National Cancer Institute in Bethesda, Md., followed 65 patients. Those who took hydrazine sulfate and were in good physical condition before the study began lived an average of 17 weeks longer.[16]

In 1990, I called the major cancer hospitals in the country looking for some information on the crucial role of total parenteral nutrition (TPN) in cancer patients. Some 40 percent of cancer patients die from cachexia.[5] Yet many starving cancer patients are offered either no nutritional support or the standard TPN solution developed for intensive care units. The solution provides 70 percent of the calories going into the bloodstream in the form of glucose. All too often, I believe, these high-glucose solutions for cachectic cancer patients do not help as much as would TPN solutions with lower levels of glucose and higher levels of amino acids and lipids. These solutions would allow the patient to build strength and would not feed the tumor.[17]

The medical establishment may be missing the connection between sugar and its role in tumorigenesis. Consider the million-dollar positive emission tomography device, or PET scan, regarded as one of the ultimate cancer-detection tools. PET scans use radioactively labeled glucose to detect sugar-hungry tumor cells. PET scans are used to plot the progress of cancer patients and to assess whether present protocols are effective.[18]

In Europe, the "sugar feeds cancer" concept is so well accepted that oncologists, or cancer doctors, use the Systemic Cancer Multistep Therapy (SCMT) protocol. Conceived by Manfred von Ardenne in Germany in 1965, SCMT entails injecting patients with glucose to increase blood-glucose concentrations. This lowers pH values in cancer tissues via lactic acid formation. In turn, this intensifies the thermal sensitivity of the malignant tumors and also induces rapid growth of the cancer. Patients are then given whole-body hyperthermia (42 C core temperature) to further stress the cancer cells, followed by chemotherapy or radiation.[19] SCMT was tested on 103 patients with metastasized cancer or recurrent primary tumors in a clinical phase-I study at the Von Ardenne Institute of Applied Medical Research in Dresden, Germany. Five-year survival rates in SCMT-treated patients increased by 25 to 50 percent, and the complete rate of tumor regression increased by 30 to 50 percent.[20] The protocol induces rapid growth of the cancer, then treats the tumor with toxic therapies for a dramatic improvement in outcome.

The irrefutable role of glucose in the growth and metastasis of cancer cells can enhance many therapies. Some of these include diets designed with the glycemic index in mind to regulate increases in blood glucose, hence selectively starving the cancer cells; low-glucose TPN solutions; avocado extract to inhibit glucose uptake in cancer cells; hydrazine sulfate to inhibit gluconeogenesis in cancer cells; and SCMT.

A female patient in her 50s, with lung cancer, came to our clinic, having been given a death sentence by her Florida oncologist. She was cooperative and understood the connection between nutrition and cancer. She changed her diet considerably, leaving out 90 percent of the sugar she used to eat. She found that wheat bread and oat cereal now had their own wild sweetness, even without added sugar. With appropriately restrained medical therapy—including high-dose radiation targeted to tumor sites and fractionated chemotherapy, a technique that distributes the normal one large weekly chemo dose into a 60-hour infusion lasting days—a good attitude and an optimal nutrition program, she beat her terminal lung cancer. I saw her the other day, five years later and still disease-free, probably looking better than the doctor who told her there was no hope.

Patrick Quillin, Ph.D., R.D., C.N.S., is director of nutrition for Cancer Treatment Centers of America in Tulsa, Okla., and author of Beating Cancer With Nutrition (Nutrition Times Press, 1998).

Printed with permission from Penton Media

Cancers Sweet Tooth by Patrick Quillin

Nutrition Science News, April 2000

References

1. Warburg O. On the origin of cancer cells. Science 1956 Feb;123:309-14.

2. Volk T, et al. pH in human tumor xenografts: effect of intravenous administration of glucose. Br J Cancer 1993 Sep;68(3):492-500.

3. 3.Digirolamo M. Diet and cancer: markers, prevention and treatment. New York: Plenum Press; 1994. p 203.

4. Leeper DB, et al. Effect of i.v. glucose versus combined i.v. plus oral glucose on human tumor extracellular pH for potential sensitization to thermoradiotherapy. Int J Hyperthermia 1998 May-Jun;14(3):257-69.

5. Rossi-Fanelli F, et al. Abnormal substrate metabolism and nutritional strategies in cancer management. JPEN J Parenter Enteral Nutr 1991 Nov-Dec;15(6):680-3.

6. Grant JP. Proper use and recognized role of TPN in the cancer patient. Nutrition 1990 Jul-Aug;6(4 Suppl):6S-7S, 10S.

7. Brand-Miller J, et al. The glucose revolution. Newport (RI) Marlowe and Co.; 1999.

8. Mooradian AD, et al. Glucotoxicity: potential mechanisms. Clin Geriatr Med 1999 May;15(2):255.

9. Hoehn, SK, et al. Complex versus simple carbohydrates and mammary tumors in mice. Nutr Cancer 1979;1(3):27.

10. Santisteban GA, et al. Glycemic modulation of tumor tolerance in a mouse model of breast cancer. Biochem Biophys Res Commun 1985 Nov 15;132(3):1174-9.

11. Sanchez A, et al. Role of sugars in human neutrophilic phagocytosis. Am J Clin Nutr 1973 Nov;26(11):1180-4.

12. Moerman CJ, et al. Dietary sugar intake in the aetiology of biliary tract cancer. Int J Epidemiol 1993 Apr;22(2):207-14.

13. Seeley S. Diet and breast cancer: the possible connection with sugar consumption. Med Hypotheses 1983 Jul;11(3):319-27.

14. Board M, et al. High Km glucose-phosphorylating (glucokinase) activities in a range of tumor cell lines and inhibition of rates of tumor growth by the specific enzyme inhibitor mannoheptulose. Cancer Res 1995 Aug 1;55(15):3278-85.

15. Chlebowski RT, et al. Hydrazine sulfate in cancer patients with weight loss. A placebo-controlled clinical experience. Cancer 1987 Feb 1;59(3):406-10.

16. Chlebowski RT, et al. Hydrazine sulfate influence on nutritional status and survival in non-small-cell lung cancer. J Clin Oncol 1990 Jan;8(1):9-15.

17. American College of Physicians. Parenteral nutrition in patients receiving cancer chemotherapy. Ann Intern Med 1989 May;110(9):734.

18. Gatenby RA. Potential role of FDG-PET imaging in understanding tumor-host interaction. J Nucl Med 1995 May;36(5):893-9.

19. von Ardenne M. Principles and concept 1993 of the Systemic Cancer Multi-step Therapy (SCMT). Extreme whole-body hyperthermia using the infra-red-A technique IRATHERM 2000—selective thermosensitisation by hyperglycemia—circulatory back-up by adapted hyperoxemia. Strahlenther Onkol 1994 Oct;170(10):581-9.

20. Steinhausen D, et al. Evaluation of systemic tolerance of 42.0 degrees C infrared-A whole-body hyperthermia in combination with hyperglycemia and hyperoxemia. A Phase-I study. Strahlenther Onkol 1994 Jun;170(6):322-34.

Milk and the Cancer Connection

Hans R. Larsen, MSc ChE

On January 23, 1998 researchers at the Harvard Medical School released a major study providing conclusive evidence that IGF-1 is a potent risk factor for prostate cancer. Should you be concerned? Yes, you certainly should, particularly if you drink milk produced in the United States.

IGF-1 or insulin-like growth factor 1 is an important hormone which is produced in the liver and body tissues. It is a polypeptide and consists of 70 amino acids linked together. All mammals produce IGF-1 molecules very similar in structure and human and bovine IGF-1 are completely identical. IGF-1 acquired its name because it has insulin-like activity in fat (adipose) tissue and has a structure which is very similar to that of proinsulin.

The body's production of IGF-1 is regulated by the human growth hormone and peaks at puberty. IGF-1 production declines with age and is only about half the adult value at the age of 70 years. IGF-1 is a very powerful hormone which has profound effects even though its concentration in the blood serum is only about 200 ng/mL or 0.2 millionth of a gram per milliliter (1-4).

IGF-1 and Cancer

IGF-1 is known to stimulate the growth of both normal and cancerous cells (2, 5). In 1990 researchers at Stanford University reported that IGF-1 promotes the growth of prostate cells (2). This was followed by the discovery that IGF-1 accelerates the growth of breast cancer cells (6-8).

In 1995 researchers at the National Institutes of Health reported that IGF-1 plays a central role in the progression of many childhood cancers and in the growth of tumors in breast cancer, small cell lung cancer, melanoma, and cancers of the pancreas and prostate(9). In September 1997 an international team of researchers reported the first epidemiological evidence that high IGF-1 concentrations are closely linked to an increased risk of prostate cancer (10).

Other researchers provided evidence of IGF-1's link to breast and colon cancers (10, 11). The January 1998 report by the Harvard researchers confirmed the link between IGF-1 levels in the blood and the risk of prostate cancer.

The effects of IGF-1 concentrations on prostate cancer risk were found to be astoundingly large—much higher than for any other known risk factor. Men having an IGF-1 level between approximately 300 and 500 ng/mL were found to have more than *four times the risk of developing prostate cancer* than did men with a level between 100 and 185 ng/mL.

The detrimental effect of high IGF-1 levels was particularly pronounced in men over 60 years of age. In this age group men with the highest levels of IGF-1 were eight times more likely to develop prostate cancer than men with low levels. The elevated IGF-1 levels were found to be present several years before an actual diagnosis of prostate cancer was made (12).

The evidence of a strong link between cancer risk and a high level of IGF-1 is now indisputable. The question is why do some people have high levels while others do not? Is it all genetically ordained or could it be that diet or some other outside factor influences IGF-1 levels? Dr. Samuel Epstein of the University of Illinois is one scientist who strongly believes so.

His 1996 article in the International Journal of Health Sciences clearly warned of the danger of high levels of IGF-1 contained in milk from cows injected with synthetic bovine growth hormone (rBGH). He postulated that IGF-1 in rBGH-milk could be a potential risk factor for breast and gastrointestinal cancers (13).

The Milk Connection

Bovine growth hormone was first synthesized in the early 1980s using genetic engineering techniques (recombinant DNA biotechnology). Small scale industry-sponsored trials showed that it was effective in increasing milk yields by an average of 14 per cent if injected into cows every two weeks.

In 1985 the Food and Drug Administration (FDA) in the United States approved the sale of milk from cows treated with rBGH (also known as BST) in large scale veterinary trials and in 1993 approved commercial sale of milk from rBGH-injected cows (13-16). At the same time the FDA prohibited the special labelling of the milk so as to make it impossible for the consumer to decide whether or not to purchase it (13).

Concerns about the safety of milk from BST-treated cows were raised as early as 1988 by scientists in both England and the United States (14, 15, 17-22). One of the main concerns is the high levels of IGF-1 found in milk from treated cows;

estimates vary from twice as high to 10 times higher than in normal cow's milk (13, 14, 23). There is also concern that the IGF-1 found in treated milk is much more potent than that found in regular milk because it seems to be bound less firmly to its accompanying proteins (13).

The concerns were vigorously attacked by consultants paid by Monsanto, the major manufacturer of rBGH. In an article published in the Journal of the American Medical Association in August 1990 the consultants claimed that BST-milk was entirely safe for human consumption (16, 24).

They pointed out that BST-milk contains no more IGF-1 than does human breast milk—a somewhat curious argument as very few grown-ups continue to drink mother's milk throughout their adult life. They also claimed that IGF-1 would be completely broken down by digestive enzymes and therefore would have no biological activity in humans (16).

Other researchers disagree with this claim and have warned that IGF-1 may not be totally digested and that some of it could indeed make its way into the colon and cross the intestinal wall into the bloodstream. This is of special concern in the case of very young infants and people who lack digestive enzymes or suffer from protein-related allergies (13, 14, 20, 22, 25).

Researchers at the FDA reported in 1990 that IGF-1 is not destroyed by pasteurization and that pasteurization actually increases its concentration in BST-milk. They also confirmed that undigested protein could indeed cross the intestinal wall in humans and cited tests which showed that oral ingestion of IGF-1 produced a significant increase in the growth of a group of male rats—a finding dismissed earlier by the Monsanto scientists (25).

The most important aspect of these experiments is that they show th*at IGF-1 can indeed enter the blood stream from the intestines*—at least in rats.

Unfortunately, essentially all the scientific data used by the FDA in the approval process was provided by the manufacturers of rBGH and much of it has since been questioned by independent scientists. The effect of IGF-1 in rBGH-milk on human health has never actually been tested and in March 1991 researchers at the National Institutes of Health admitted that it was not known whether IGF-1 in milk from treated cows could have a local effect on the esophagus, stomach or intestines (26, 27).

Whether IGF-1 in milk is digested and broken down into its constituent amino acids or whether it enters the intestine intact is a crucial factor. No human studies have been done on this, but recent research has shown that a very similar hormone, Epidermal Growth Factor, is protected against digestion when ingested in the presence of casein, a main component of milk (13, 23, 28).

Thus there is a distinct possibility that IGF-1 in milk could also avoid digestion and make its way into the intestine where it could promote colon cancer (13, 22). It is also conceivable that it could cross the intestinal wall in sufficient amounts to increase the blood level of IGF-1 significantly and thereby increase the risk of breast and prostate cancers (13, 14).

The Bottom Line

Despite assurances from the FDA and industry-paid consultants there are now just too many serious questions surrounding the use of milk from cows treated with synthetic growth hormone to allow its continued sale. Bovine growth hormone is banned in Australia, New Zealand and Japan.

The European Union has maintained its moratorium on the use of rBGH and milk products from BST-treated cows are not sold in countries within the Union. Canada has also so far resisted pressure from the United States and the biotechnology lobby to approve the use of rBGH commercially.

In light of the serious concerns about the safety of human consumption of milk from BST-treated cows consumers must maintain their vigilance to ensure that European and Canadian governments continue to resist the pressure to approve rBGH and that the FDA in the United States moves immediately to ban rBGH-milk or at least allow its labeling so that consumers can protect themselves against the very real cancer risks posed by IGF-1.

From International Health News (Reprinted with permission from Hans Larsen)

(http://www.yourhealthbase.com/milk_cancer.htm)

References

1.   *Wilson, Jean D. and Foster, Daniel W., eds. Williams Textbook of Endocrinology, 8th edition, London, W.B. Saunders Company, 1992, pp. 1096-1106*

2. Cohen, Pinchas, et al. *Insulin-like growth factors (IGFs), IGF receptors, and IGF-binding proteins in primary cultures of prostate epithelial cells.* Journal of Clinical Endocrinology and Metabolism, Vol. 73, No. 2, 1991, pp. 401-07

3. Rudman, Daniel, et al. *Effects of human growth hormone in men over 60 years old.* New England Journal of Medicine, Vol. 323, July 5, 1990, pp. 1-6

4. LeRoith, Derek, moderator. *Insulin-like growth factors in health and disease.* Annals of Internal Medicine, Vol. 116, May 15, 1992, pp. 854-62

5. Rosenfeld, R.G., et al. *Insulin-like growth factor binding proteins in neoplasia (meeting abstract).* Hormones and Growth Factors in Development and Neoplasia, Fogarty International Conference, June 26-28, 1995, Bethesda, MD, 1995, p. 24

6. Lippman, Marc E. *The development of biological therapies for breast cancer.* Science, Vol. 259, January 29, 1993, pp. 631-32

7. Papa, Vincenzo, et al. *Insulin-like growth factor-I receptors are overexpressed and predict a low risk in human breast cancer.* Cancer Research, Vol. 53, 1993, pp. 3736-40

8. Stoll, B.A. *Breast cancer: further metabolic-endocrine risk markers?* British Journal of Cancer, Vol. 76, No. 12, 1997, pp. 1652-54

9. LeRoith, Derek, et al. *The role of the insulin-like growth factor-I receptor in cancer.* Annals New York Academy of Sciences, Vol. 766, September 7, 1995, pp. 402-08

10. Mantzoros, C.S., et al. *Insulin-like growth factor 1 in relation to prostate cancer and benign prostatic hyperplasia.* British Journal of Cancer, Vol. 76, No. 9, 1997, pp. 1115-18

11. Cascinu, S., et al. *Inhibition of tumor cell kinetics and serum insulin growth factor I levels by octreotide in colorectal cancer patients.* Gastroenterology, Vol. 113, September 1997, pp. 767-72

12. Chan, June M., et al. *Plasma insulin-like growth factor I and prostate cancer risk: a prospective study.* Science, Vol. 279, January 23, 1998, pp. 563-66

13. *Epstein, Samuel S. Unlabeled milk from cows treated with biosynthetic growth hormones: a case of regulatory abdication. International Journal of Health Services, Vol. 26, No. 1, 1996, pp. 173-85*

14. *Epstein, Samuel S. Potential public health hazards of biosynthetic milk hormones. International Journal of Health Services, Vol. 20, No. 1, 1990, pp. 73-84*

15. *Epstein, Samuel S. Questions and answers on synthetic bovine growth hormones. International Journal of Health Services, Vol. 20, No. 4, 1990, pp. 573-82*

16. *Daughaday, William H. and Barbano, David M. Bovine somatotropin supplementation of dairy cows—Is the milk safe? Journal of the American Medical Association, Vol. 264, August 22/29, 1990, pp. 1003-05*

17. *Brunner, Eric. Safety of bovine somatotropin. The Lancet, September 10, 1988, p. 629 (letter to the editor)*

18. *Kronfeld, D.S., et al. Bovine somatotropin. Journal of the American Medical Association, Vol. 265, March 20, 1991, pp. 1389-91 (letters to the editor)*

19. *Rubin, Andrew L. and Goodman, Mark. Milk safety. Science, Vol. 264, May 13, 1993, pp. 889-90 (letters to the editor)*

20. *Challacombe, D.N., et al. Safety of milk from cows treated with bovine somatotrophin. The Lancet, Vol. 344, September 17, 1994, pp. 815-17 (letters to the editor)*

21. *Coghlan, Andy. Milk hormone data bottled up for years. New Scientist, October 22, 1994, p. 4*

22. *Coghlan, Andy. Arguing till the cows come home. New Scientist, October 29, 1994, pp. 14-15*

23. *Mepham, T.B., et al. Safety of milk from cows treated with bovine somatotrophin. The Lancet, Vol. 344, July 16, 1994, pp. 197-98 (letter to the editor)*

24. *Grossman, Charles J. Genetic engineering and the use of bovine somatotropin. Journal of the American Medical Association, Vol. 264, August 22/29, 1990, p. 1028 (editorial)*

25. *Juskevich, Judith C. and Guyer, C. Greg. Bovine growth hormone: human food safety evaluation. Science, Vol. 249, August 24, 1990, pp. 875-84*

26. *Mepham, T.B. Bovine somatotrophin and public health. British Medical Journal, Vol. 302, March 2, 1991, pp. 483-84*

27. *NIH technology assessment conference statement on bovine somatotropin. Journal of the American Medical Association, Vol. 265, March 20, 1991, pp. 1423-25*

28. Playford, R.J., et al. Effect of luminal growth factor preservation on intestinal growth. The Lancet, Vol. 341, April 3, 1993, pp. 843-48

The Six Dangers of Common Beef, and How to Avoid Them

By Dr. Joseph Mercola
with Rachael Droege

www.mercola.com

Beef is a mainstay of the traditional American dinner. Many even eat it for lunch or a late night snack. Its many forms show up at summer barbecues, holiday feasts, workday dinners, and just about anywhere that people are eating. In fact, Americans eat more meat than any other population in the world, with the typical American eating over 60 pounds of beef a year. Which brings me to my point—much of this beef, the vast majority of it by far, is filled with harmful additives and is raised in such a way that it at best provides little more for your body than something to fill your stomach, and at worst is contributing to the degeneration of your health.

Think about it—do you really know where your prime rib or hamburger meat came from? Where did the animal live? How was it raised? What did it eat? Was it healthy or diseased? Perhaps you'd rather not think about it because you have an intuitive feeling that the answer would not be pretty.

Most Commercial Cattle are Fed Grains

As more and more Americans realize the importance of eliminating or reducing grains in their diets, beef is likely to become an increasingly popular substitution. However, since nearly all cattle are grain-fed before slaughter, if you eat most traditionally raised beef it will typically worsen your omega-6:omega-3 ratio.

According to a study published in The European Journal of Clinical Nutrition, livestock that are fed on grain have more omega-6 fat, which may promote heart disease, and less omega-3 fat, which is beneficial for cardiac health, than both wild animals and grass-fed livestock.

It is therefore much to your advantage to eat grass-fed beef, but you must also be careful as many stores will advertise beef as grass-fed when it really isn't. They do this as ALL cattle are grass-fed, but the key is what they are fed in the months prior to being processed. You will need to call the person who actually raised the cows, NOT the store manager, to find out the truth.

The least expensive way to obtain authentic grass-fed beef would be to find a farmer who is growing the beef who you can trust and buy a half a side of beef from him. This way you save the shipping and also receive a reduced rate on the meat. Alternatively, you can order authentic grass-fed beef from our site.

An inexpensive, yet effective, way to determine if the beef is really from a grass-fed animal is to purchase the ground beef. Slowly cook the beef till done and drain and collect all the fat. Grass-fed beef is very high in omega-3 fats and will be relatively thin compared to traditionally prepared ground beef. It will also be a liquid at room temperature as it has very few saturated fats, which are mostly solid at room temperature.

Hormones

Most traditionally raised beef calves go from 80 pounds to 1,200 pounds in a period of about 14 months. This is no natural feat. Along with enormous quantities of grain (usually corn) and protein supplements, calves are fed or implanted with various drugs and hormones to, as the beef industry says, "promote efficient growth."

Any combination of the natural hormones estradiol, progesterone, and testosterone, and the synthetic hormones zeranol and trenbolone acetate may be given to cattle. Another hormone, melengesterol acetate, may also be added to feed to "improve weight gain and feed efficiency."

Measurable amounts of hormones in traditionally raised beef are transferred to humans, and some scientists believe that human consumption of estrogen from hormone-fed beef can result in cancer, premature puberty and falling sperm counts.

Antibiotics

About nine million pounds of antibiotic feed additives are used annually in the cattle-raising process. Many people don't realize that the largest use of antibiotics in the United States is to feed to animals, often so that they will gain more weight, but also to prevent disease outbreaks that could easily fester since the animals are raised in such crowded conditions.

This routine antibiotic use is contributing to the growing problem of antibiotic resistance in humans. Animals raised in natural environments, not the traditional "factory farms," rarely require antibiotics. You may be able to find antibiotic-free beef in your local health food store, but be sure to be certain that it is grass-fed as well.

Along with antibiotics, traditionally raised cattle are given various vaccines and other drugs. The following is just one recommended course of care for a whole herd of cattle as shown on Pfizer.com:

- CattleMaster 4+VL5: a 4-way viral plus 5-way leptospirosis vaccine and vibriosis protection
- UltraChoice 8: a vaccine to prevent clostridial diseases
- Dectomax Pour-On or Dectomax Injectable: drugs to prevent and treat internal and external parasites
- ScourGuard 3®(K)/C: a vaccine to prevent calf scours

Irradiation

Some commercial beef is irradiated, which means it has been treated with gamma rays produced by the radioactive material, cobalt 60, or electricity to kill bacteria. The effects of long-term consumption of irradiated food products remain to be seen.

This issue is virtually the same issue as with milk. Once milk is pasteurized to "protect" us, it is seriously damaged and actually causes more harm than good for most who drink it. However, if milk is consumed in its real raw form, then it is typically an amazing health-producing food for most who consume it.

If you value your long-term health, I strongly encourage you to avoid irradiated meat. All meats will not be irradiated, so your best bet is to purchase non-irradiated meat.

Many may not be aware that school districts have the option of purchasing irradiated beef for their lunch programs, and parental notification is not required. If you are a parent you can work with your school district to discourage the use of irradiated foods, or at the very least contact them to find out whether irradiated beef is being served in your child's school cafeteria.

The following Web site has more information on how to work with your school district to stop the purchase of irradiated foods: www.safelunch.org.

You can also contact your representative and senators today to urge them not to support irradiated food in school lunches.

Environmental Problems

Alongside the dangers that traditionally raised beef pose to your health are the dangers they pose to your environment. Substantial areas of forests, particularly the rain forests of Central America and the Amazon, are being cleared to make way for cattle. And in the United States, cattle production is a major source of environmental pollution.

Among the most severe problems are water pollution from the nearly 1 billion tons of organic waste produced by cattle each year and the enormous amounts of petro-chemical fertilizers used to produce feed crops, and air pollution—waste and waste treatment methods of grain-fed cattle are responsible for producing a significant portion of carbon dioxide, methane, and nitrous oxide (the three major gases that are largely responsible for global warming), along with other harmful gasses.

Inhumane Treatment of Cattle

Traditionally raised cattle are treated as commodities and are deprived of some of the most basic requirements of life—fresh air, space and normal social interaction. Along with the health benefits of the grass-fed beef on our site, you can rest assured that the animals are raised in their natural environment—a green pasture.

Reprinted with Permission from mercola.com

Cited from http://www.mercola.com/2003/dec/20/beef_dangers.htm

A Good Nights Sleep May Help Prevent Cancer

Matthew J. Loop, D.C.

Concentrating your focus on your sleep habits could help to prevent cancer, believe it or not! It has been known for years that how well you sleep may drastically alter the stability of hormones in the human body. Shifts from balanced hormones can disturb your sleep/wake cycle, also referred to as the circadian rhythm. An altered circadian rhythm may affect how cancer progresses through shifts in hormones like melatonin, which the brain manufactures during sleep.

Investigative research discovered in *Brain Behavior Immunology October 2003* suggested having a normal circadian rhythm may be vital in order for your body to protect against cancer. It further suggested sleep/wake rhythms that are thrown off due to stress or other issues may encourage the growth of cancer.

The antioxidant melatonin has properties that aide in the suppression of destructive free radicals in the body and it decreases the manufacturing of estrogen, which can trigger cancer. When circadian rhythm's become upset, it may create a smaller amount melatonin and therefore may have a decreased ability to protect against cancer. Light exposure throughout the evening can also lessen melatonin levels, hence making it imperative to sleep in total darkness to reduce the risk of cancer. An additional association between cancer and an upset circadian rhythm deals with the hormone cortisol, which regularly reaches its highest levels at dawn then drops during the day. Cortisol is only one of numerous hormones that assist in regulating immune system function, including the activity of immune cells called natural-killer cells that aide the body fighting cancer.

One more mechanism that might be connected to the cancer/sleep relationship is the hormone insulin. Scientific researchers from the University of Chicago have time and again shown that
a lack of sleep will culminate in an elevated rate of diabetes due to heightened insulin resistance, and insulin has been obviously connected to cancer in studies held prior.

Sleep is extremely important. It has continuously been shown that not enough rest will result in elevated rates of cancer and diabetes, while optimizing your sleep may dramatically slow down aging in general. Below are some tips and guidelines that will allow you to maximize and get the proper amount of sleep your body requires.

- *Absolutely no TV right before bed.* TV, or any light for that matter, can disturb your circadian rhythm and your pineal gland's manufacturing of melatonin and seratonin.

- *Our body's natural biorhythm is to experience sleep roughly around 10 P.M. to 6 A.M.* The lights should be out by 10 P.M. and you should "rise-and-shine" by 6 A.M. Those who find this difficult, be aware that individuals normally followed this pattern before the electricity was ever conceived.

- *Avoid electro-magnetic fields (EMFs) in the bedroom.* A few examples are cell phones, microwaves, TV's, computers, some alarm clocks, etc. All of these can disturb the pineal gland and the manufacture of melatonin and seratonin, as well as contributing to other negative effects as well.

- *Avoid late-night and before bedtime snacks, especially grains and sugars.* These will elevate blood sugar and deter sleep. After awhile, when blood sugar drops too low, you may wake up and have trouble falling asleep again.

- *Lessen your mental activity after dinner.* Journaling might help in this process by allowing you to put your worries on paper and get them out of your mind.

- *Plan for the following day,* like formulating what you intend to get done, so it's not on your mind all night.

- *Avoid alcohol at all costs.* Even though alcohol will make individuals drowsy, the effect doesn't last that long and people will frequently wake up many hours later and be incapable of getting back to sleep. Consuming alcohol will also keep you from experiencing the deep stages of sleep, where the human body performs much of its healing.

- *Soak in a hot bath for up to an hour with relaxing fragrances* (vanilla, sandalwood, lavender) 30 minutes prior to retiring. Use the bath to let go of your daily stress, include soothing lights and music and massage your body with oils.

- *Your bed should be used for only sleep and sex.* Even reading should be done elsewhere, unless it has a calming effect, such as spiritual literature.

- *Make sure to turn all lights off.* Rest on your back or side and pay attention to the way your body feels as well as to your breathing.

- *Try reciting a mantra for five minutes.* This could be some sort of favorite sound or prayer that you recite continuously.

- *I recommend reducing or avoiding as many drugs as possible.* Numerous medications, both prescription and over-the-counter might have effects on sleep as listed under side effects.

- *If you have difficulty sleeping in your bed, try another area in your house.*

- *Refrain from using loud alarm clocks.* It is extremely stressful on the body to be awoken abruptly. If you are regularly getting enough sleep, they should be unnecessary. Sun alarm clocks or ones that have a progressive nature sound are the best ones have. The Sun Alarm can be purchased at www.mercola.com.

Fluoridated Water and the Link to Cancer

Former Harvard University dental student, Dr. Elise Bassin's findings finally became public recently and it could be big trouble to fluoride proponents, and, in particular, Bassin's former college advisor and current boss, Chester Douglass, who chairs the Oral Health Policy and Epidemiology department at Harvard University. Douglass says her study was a subset of his own $1.3 million, 15-year study funded by the National Institutes of Health that *debunked* any connection between fluoride and cancer.

Many people are unaware that Douglass is also compensated as an editor of the Colgate Oral Care Report, a newsletter supported by one of the leading makers of *fluoride toothpaste* in the world

Dr. Bassin's study investigated young boys who drink fluoridated water. Fluoridated water is supposedly considered safe based on federal regulations but he found a *five times greater risk* of developing osteosarcoma, the most common kind of bone cancer.

Since children are being harmed by the fluoride toxicity in their teeth and bones, there is plenty of reason to remove it from your home water supply.

Reprinted with kind permission of Springer Science and Business Media

Age-specific Fluoride Exposure in Drinking Water and Osteosarcoma (United States) by Elise B. Bassin

Cancer Causes and Control May 2006: Volume 17; Number 4; pages 421-428

How Is Antibiotic Use Linked to Cancer?

A new investigative study points to the fact that heavy use of antibiotics during childhood elevates the likelihood of developing cancer that affects the body's lymphatic system, referred to as non-Hodgkin's lymphoma (NHL).

The Remarkable Correlation

Experts reviewed information from the Scandinavian Lymphoma Etiology study, which compared over 3,000 patients with NHL with a similar number of healthy patients. There was a "striking" association between antibiotic use and NHL for all subtypes of the disease, especially for those who had been given antibiotics greater than 10 times as children.

These findings may indicate that the rising use of antibiotics in the 20th century may also clarify the rise in NHL cases. Scientific researchers state it is unknown whether antibiotic therapy caused the NHL, or if antibiotics are just more likely to be taken by those susceptible to developing NHL.

NSAIDs have Similar Correlation

An elevated risk of NHL for intense users of non-steroidal anti-inflammatory drugs (NSAIDs) was also shown to have correlative findings. Within this realm are ibuprofen drugs such as Advil and Motrin.

Reprinted with permission from Oxford University Press

Medication Use and Risk of Non-Hodgkin's Lymphoma by Ellen T. Chang

American Journal of Epidemiology November 15, 2005; 162 (10): 965-974

The Drug Ritalin Implicated in Increasing Cancer Risks

Around 30 million prescriptions for the drug Ritalin, and similar drugs to treat attention deficit hyperactivity disorder (ADHD), were written in 2004 in the United States. An astonishing 23 million prescriptions were for children alone. These drugs remain some of the most controversial and are included within the most widely prescribed medications worldwide.

The most recent episode in the dispute over the safety of ADHD drugs is The Food and Drug Administration's (FDA) inquiry regarding an association between Ritalin and cancer—based on a University of Texas scientific study.

The results found the chromosomes of 12 children who had taken Ritalin for three months were damaged.

And while the Texas researchers claimed their study was far too small to prompt the parents of attention deficit patients to abandon Ritalin and may contain some methodology flaws, the FDA, National Institutes of Health (NIH) and the Environmental Protection Agency found the results merited public concern and further study.

Possible Label Changes down the line?

Recent reports about Ritalin's potential connection to cancer comes in juxtaposition with another health issue surrounding the class of ADHD medications known as methylphenidates. Ritalin is classified within this category.

In effect, the FDA has been taking into consideration label changes to all methylphenidates due to possible psychiatric events and cardiovascular side effects. An earlier review revealed:

- Thirty-six psychiatric events (hallucinations and suicide ideation) for Concerta, compared to 16 for Ritalin and other methylphenidates.

- Concerta had 20 cardiovascular event reports; other methylphenidates had four.

Labeling changes may not be the answer, according to many critics.

According to the director of the child and adolescent psychiatry clinic at Jackson Memorial Hospital and an associate professor of psychiatry at the University of

Miami School of Medicine, labeling is an oversimplification of the problem and doesn't address the many other problems that are affecting the outcome.

Reprinted with permission from Elsevier

Cancer Letters Volume 230, Issue 2, December 18, 2005, Pg 284-291

Cytogenetic effects of children treated with Methylphenidate by Randa A. El-Zein

Snack Chips, French Fries Show Highest Levels of Known Carcinogen

Popular American brands of snack chips and French fries contain disturbingly high levels of acrylamide, according to new laboratory tests commissioned by the Center for Science in the Public Interest (CSPI). The tests were conducted by the same Swedish government scientists that two months ago first discovered the cancer-causing chemical in certain fried and baked starchy foods. CSPI's tests included several popular brands of snack chips, taco shells, French fries, and breakfast cereals—the kinds of foods that were initially shown to have some of the highest acrylamide levels.

Today is the first day of a three-day closed meeting in Geneva of experts convened by the World Health Organization (WHO) to discuss the health ramifications of the acrylamide discovery, which has since been confirmed by the British, Swiss, and Norwegian governments. The United States Food and Drug Administration (FDA) though, has been standing on the sidelines of what is fast becoming a major global debate, according to CSPI, which today called on the agency to treat acrylamide with greater seriousness.

"The FDA has been strangely silent about acrylamide," CSPI executive director Michael F. Jacobson said. "It should be advising consumers to avoid or cut back on the most contaminated and least nutritious foods while more testing is done across the food supply. The FDA also should be intensively investigating ways of preventing the formation of this carcinogen."

Fast-food French fries showed the highest levels of acrylamide among the foods CSPI had tested, with large orders containing 39 to 82 micrograms. One-ounce portions of Pringles potato crisps contained about 25 micrograms, with corn-based Fritos and Tostitos containing half that amount or less. Regular and Honey Nut Cheerios contained 6 or 7 micrograms of the carcinogenic substance. Among the findings:

Acrylamide in Foods: Micrograms per Serving	
Water, 8 oz., EPA limit	0.12
Boiled Potatoes, 4 oz.	<3
Old El Paso Taco Shells, 3, 1.1oz.	1

Acrylamide in Foods: Micrograms per Serving	
Ore Ida French Fries (uncooked), 3 oz.	5
Ore Ida French Fries (baked), 3 oz.	28
Honey Nut Cheerios, 1 oz.	6
Cheerios, 1 oz.	7
Tostitos Tortilla Chips, 1 oz.	5
Fritos Corn Chips, 1 oz.	11
Pringles Potato Crisps, 1 oz.	25
Wendy's French Fries, Biggie, 5.6 oz.	39
KFC Potato Wedges, Jumbo, 6.2 oz.	52
Burger King French Fries, large, 5.7 oz.	59
McDonald's French Fries, large, 6.2 oz.	82

The amount of acrylamide in a large order of fast-food French fries is at least 300 times more than what the U.S. Environmental Protection Agency allows in a glass of water. Acrylamide is sometimes used in water-treatment facilities.

"I estimate that acrylamide causes several thousand cancers per year in Americans," said Clark University research professor, Dale Hattis. Hattis, an expert in risk analysis, based his estimate on standard EPA projections of risks from animal studies and limited sampling of acrylamide levels in Swedish and American foods.

Acrylamide forms as a result of unknown chemical reactions during high-temperature baking or frying. Raw or even boiled potatoes test negative for the chemical. CSPI today urged the FDA to inform the public of the risks from acrylamide in different foods, and to work with industry and academia to understand how acrylamide is formed and how to prevent its formation.

"There has long been reason for Americans to eat less greasy French fries and snack chips," Jacobson said. "Acrylamide is yet another reason to eat less of those foods."

A California attorney has formally demanded that McDonald's and Burger King place a cancer warning on their French fries, as required by the state's Proposition

65. Burger King faces a legal deadline of late June and McDonald's of early July to respond.

Reprinted with permission from the *Center for Science in the Public Interest (CSPI)*, June 25, 2002

New Tests Confirm Acrylamide in American Foods by CSPI

Cited from http://www.cspinet.org/new/200206251.html

Reduce Your Risk of Cancer with Sunlight Exposure

By William B. Grant, Ph.D.
SUNARC

www.mercola.com

With all of the publicity that UV radiation (UVR) is an important cause of skin cancer, premature skin aging and cataract formation, one might think that avoidance of UVR would be the best policy. Not so fast. If protection against UVR were the most important thing, all humans would have very dark skin, since the melanin in dark skin protects against skin cancer and premature skin aging.

Skin pigmentation becomes paler the closer one's ancestors lived to the polar-regions, evidently to balance cutaneous production of vitamin D with protection against free radicals and DNA damage from UVR [Jablonski and Chaplin, 2000]. In addition, even a cursory look at the geographic variation in cancer mortality rates in the United States [Devesa et al., 1999] indicates that some environmental factor has to explain why mortality rates for a number of internal cancers are approximately twice as high in northeastern, highly-urbanized states than in southwestern, more rural states.

Diet and smoking are, of course, important risk factors for many types of cancer [Doll and Peto, 1981]. But in order for diet to explain the geographic variation in cancer rates, Americans would need to be eating drastically different diets by region. However, anyone who has travelled throughout the United States knows that the food choices do not vary much anywhere in the contiguous 48 states.

The Risk of Cancer Lessens With More Sun Exposure

The key to understanding this geographic pattern was provided by Cedric and Frank Garland in 1980 [Garland and Garland, 1980]. They reasoned that sunlight, through the production of vitamin D, reduced the risk of colon cancer in the sunny areas compared to that in the darker areas. They performed an ecologic study of annual solar irradiance versus colon cancer mortality rates and found a strong inverse correlation, i.e. the more sunlight, the less cancer. (An ecologic study treats entire populations defined geographically as entities, with values for disease outcome and environmental or dietary factors averaged for each entity.)

Their paper received little notice at first, perhaps because UVR was commonly associated with skin cancer, perhaps because the ecologic approach was falling out of favor [Doll and Peto, 1981]. Undaunted, they extended their work through the use of stored serum 25-hydroxyvitamin D (25(OH)D)—the common form of circulating vitamin D—values for another purpose along with a determination of colorectal cancer incidence among the serum donors, finding a significant inverse correlation between 25(OH)D and colorectal cancer rates [Garland et al., 1985]. The list of cancers for which ultraviolet B (UVB) (290-315 nm) and vitamin D is protective was extended through a variety of observational epidemiologic studies by the end of the 1990s to include breast, ovarian and prostate cancer and non-Hodgkin's lymphoma [Grant, 2002b].

How Vitamin D Reduces the Risk of Cancer

The mechanisms by which vitamin D reduces the risk of cancer are fairly well understood. They include enhancing calcium absorption (in the case of colorectal cancer) [Lamprecht and Lipkin, 2003], inducing cell differentiation, increasing cancer cell apoptosis or death, reducing metastasis and proliferation, and reducing angiogenesis [van den Bemd and Chang, 2002]. In addition, 25(OH)D downregulates parathyroid hormone (PTH) [Chapuy et al., 1987]. Since IGF-I stimulates tumor growth and high quantities are a consequence of the standard American diet [Grant, 2002a; 2004], vitamin D can be considered one partial antidote to the American diet.

When I decided to investigate the role of UVB and vitamin D in reducing the risk of cancer, after I convinced myself that dietary factors could not explain the geographic variation of cancer mortality rates in the United States, I posed two questions to address:

- For how many cancers is UVB/vitamin D protective?

- How many Americans die prematurely each year due to inadequate levels of vitamin D?

I started with the maps of cancer mortality rates in the Atlas of Cancer Mortality [Devesa et al., 1999] and found the UVB irradiance/dose map for the United States for July 1992 made using data obtained by NASA's Total Ozone Mapping Spectrometer (TOMS) to use as a proxy for vitamin D production. In this study, I determined that UVB was inversely correlated with mortality rates for 12 types of cancer, including five types of cancer already identified plus an additional seven, and estimated that 17, 000 to 23,000 Americans died prematurely each year due to insufficient vitamin D [Grant, 2002b].

While the study was generally accepted, critics pointed out that I had ignored a number of factors that affect the risk of cancer and which could, perhaps, explain much of the variation in mortality rates. To respond to these critics, I extended the analysis by including a number of cancer risk factors for which I could find state-averaged values.

These factors included lung cancer mortality rates (an index for the adverse health effects of smoking), fraction of the population considered of Hispanic heritage (Hispanics are counted as white Americans in the Atlas), alcohol consumption rates, degree of urbanization, and fraction of the population living below the poverty level.

Sun Exposure (UVB) Protects Against 16 Types of Cancer

The new study links UVB as protective to a total of 16 types of cancer, primarily epithelial (pertaining to the surface) cancers of the digestive and reproductive systems [Grant, submitted]. Six types of cancer (breast, colon, endometrial, esophageal, ovarian, and non-Hodgkin's lymphoma) were inversely correlated to solar UVB radiation and rural residence in combination. This result strongly suggests that living in an urban environment is associated with reduced UVB exposure compared to living in a rural environment.

Another 10 types of cancer including bladder, gallbladder, gastric, pancreatic, prostate, rectal and renal were inversely correlated with UVB but not urban residence. Ten types of cancer were significantly correlated with smoking, six types with alcohol, and seven types with Hispanic heritage. Poverty status was inversely correlated with seven types of cancer. Since the results for alcohol, Hispanic heritage, and smoking for white Americans agree well with the literature [Trapido et al., 1995; Thun et al., 2002], they provide a high level of confidence in the approach and its results for UVB radiation.

Over 40,000 Americans Die Annually From Cancer Caused by Vitamin D Deficiency

From this analysis, it was estimated that 45,000 Americans die from cancer annually related to inadequate levels of vitamin D: half from UVB doses based on location, and half based on living in an urban environment with reduced solar radiation exposure.

Papers continue to appear supporting the UVB/vitamin D-cancer connection. The latest is from Norway, showing that the detection of breast, colon, and prostate cancer has a seasonal cycle correlated with vitamin D production by sunlight [Robsahm et al., 2004]. This paper is important since it shows that vitamin D effectively fights cancer even in the later stages.

How Much Vitamin D is Required to Prevent Cancer?

The amount of ingested vitamin D and/or UVB exposure required for optimal protection against cancer is still being determined. Each person responds differently to UVB exposure and oral intake of vitamin D depending on such factors as skin pigmentation, body mass index (vitamin D is fat soluble), age, condition of digestive tract, other dietary factors, etc.

Dietary vitamin D is insufficient alone to significantly reduce the risk of most cancers since the ingested amounts, up to 200 to 400 I.U. per day, are too low [Grant and Garland, in press]. Evidently, 600 to 1000 I.U per day are required to reduce the risk of vitamin-D-sensitive cancers, except possibly prostate cancer, for which population-average values of serum 25(OH)D are associated with the minimum risk [Tuohimaa et al., 2004; Grant, in press].

The current understanding is that serum 25(OH)D levels should be in the 30 to 40 ng/ml (75-100 nmol/L) range for cancer prevention and optimal health. The only way to determine one's 25(OH)D levels is through blood tests, which can be ordered through a physician or nutritionist. It should be noted that the UVB dose required to generate these levels is much less than would ordinarily be considered a risk factor for skin cancer, etc.

The time required in the sun is probably 15 to 30 minutes per day with at least hands and face exposed in the mid-latitudes during summer [Reid et al., 1986], but depends on a number of personal factors. The optimal time for solar UVB production of vitamin D may be around the middle of the day when the ratio of UVB to UVA (315-400 nm) is highest and the required exposure times are shortest.

However, this works only when the sun is elevated high enough—for the four to five darkest months of the year it is impossible to produce any vitamin D from sunlight in Boston [Webb et al., 1988]. When solar UVB is not available, one has to rely on stored vitamin D (weeks to months), artificial UVB, dietary supplements, many types of fish, or fortified foods, which now include milk and orange juice.

How Can You Protect Yourself From Inadequate Vitamin D Levels?

While the scientific results to date increasingly support the hypothesis that UVB and vitamin D reduce the risk of many types of cancer as well as many other types of disease including musculoskeletal diseases, autoimmune diseases and hypertension, it will likely be some time before the health system embraces this hypothesis and acts to recommend higher values of 25(OH)D, which would require increased UVB exposure (natural and artificial) and dietary supplements.

However, the informed individual who carefully studies the literature can very likely reduce his or her risk of cancer and a number of other diseases by careful exposure to UVB, being particularly careful to avoid any sunburning, and adequate intake of vitamin D.

More information on the protective role of UVB against breast and colorectal cancer, other cancers, and other diseases can be found at my Web site, www.sunarc.org.

William B. Grant has a Ph.D. in physics from U.C. Berkeley and has worked at the level of senior research scientist in the fields of optical and laser remote sensing of the atmosphere and atmospheric sciences at SRI International, the Jet Propulsion Laboratory, and the NASA Langley Research Center. He is the author or coauthor of over 60 articles in peer-reviewed journals, has edited two books of reprints, and contributed half a dozen chapters to other books.

He published the first paper linking diet to Alzheimer's disease and identifying the major dietary components that are risk and risk reduction factors. He has also studied the links between dietary sugars and heart disease and obesity, diet and breast, colon and prostate cancer, and UVB/vitamin D and cancer and autoimmune diseases. He recently retired from NASA and founded Sunlight, Nutrition and Health Research Center (SUNARC), where he will continue and extend his health research and educational efforts.

References

1. Chapuy MC, Chapuy P, Meunier PJ. Calcium and vitamin D supplements: effects on calcium metabolism in elderly people. Am J Clin Nutr. 1987;46:324-8.

2. Devesa SS, Grauman DJ, Blot WJ, Pennello GA, Hoover RN, Fraumeni JF Jr., Atlas of Cancer Mortality in the United States, 1950-1994. NIH Publication No. 99-4564, 1999. website (accessed March 3, 2004).

3. Doll R, Peto R. The causes of cancer: quantitative estimates of avoidable risks of cancer in the United States today. J Natl Cancer Inst. 1981; 66:1191-308.

4. Garland CF, Garland FC. Do sunlight and vitamin D reduce the likelihood of colon cancer? Int J Epidemiol. 1980;9:227-31.

5. Garland C, Shekelle RB, Barrett-Connor E, Criqui MH, Rossof AH, Paul O. Dietary vitamin D and calcium and risk of colorectal cancer: a 19-year prospective study in men. Lancet. 1985;1:307-9.

6. Grant WB. An estimate of premature cancer mortality in the United States due to inadequate doses of solar ultraviolet-B radiation, Cancer, 2002b;94:1867-75.

7. Grant WB. A multicountry ecologic study of risk and risk reduction factors for prostate cancer mortality. Eur Urol. 2004;45:371-9.

8. Grant WB. Geographic variation of prostate cancer mortality rates in the U.S.A.; implications for prostate cancer risk related to vitamin D; Int. J. Cancer, in press.

9. Grant WB, Garland CF. A critical review of studies on vitamin D in relation to colorectal cancer. Nutrition Cancer, in press.

10. Herman JR, Krotkov N, Celarier E, Larko E, Labow G. Distribution of UV radiation at the Earth's surface from TOMS-measured UV-backscattered radiances. J Geophys Res-Atmos. 1999;104:12,059-12,076. website (accessed February 25, 2004).

11. Jablonski NG, Chaplin G. The evolution of human skin coloration. J Hum Evol. 2000;39:57-106.

12. Lamprecht SA, Lipkin M. Chemoprevention of colon cancer by calcium, vitamin D and folate: molecular mechanisms. Nat Rev Cancer. 2003;3:601-14.

13. Reid IR, Gallagher DJ, Bosworth J. Prophylaxis against vitamin D deficiency in the elderly by regular sunlight exposure. Age Ageing. 1986;15:35-40.

14. Robsahm TE, Tretli S, Dahlback A, Moan J. Vitamin D(3) from sunlight may improve the prognosis of breast-, colon- and prostate cancer (Norway). Cancer Causes Control. 2004;15:149-58.

15. Thun MJ, Henley SJ, Calle EE. Tobacco use and cancer: an epidemiologic perspective for geneticists. Oncogene 2002;21:7307-25.

16. Tuohimaa P, Tenkanen L, Ahonen M, et al. Both high and low levels of blood vitamin D are associated with a higher prostate cancer risk: a longitudinal, nested case-control study in the Nordic countries. Int J Cancer. 2004;108:104-8.

17. van den Bemd GJ, Chang GT. Vitamin D and vitamin D analogs in cancer treatment. Curr Drug Targets. 2002;3:85-94.

18. Webb AR, Kline L, Holick MF. Influence of season and latitude on the cutaneous synthesis of vitamin D3: exposure to winter sunlight in Boston and Edmonton will not promote vitamin D3 synthesis in human skin. J Clin Endocrinol Metab. 1988;67:373-8.

Reprinted with Permission from mercola.com

Cited from http://www.mercola.com/2004/mar/31/cancer_sunlight.htm

Cancer Prevention Using Garlic?

Scientific researchers suggest that consuming garlic appears to defend against stomach and colon cancer. A review of 18 studies looking at those who consume garlic was conducted by Dr. Lenore Arab and colleagues at the University of North Carolina at Chapel Hill.

- Average intake of the greatest eaters of raw or cooked garlic was 18.3 grams per week, which is around six cloves.

- Based on six studies, the conclusions suggest *"high consumption of raw or cooked garlic decreases the risk of colorectal cancer from 10% to nearly 50%,"* the authors write.

- Based on four studies, the risk of developing stomach cancer was shrunk by half for those who readily ate the most garlic.

Reprinted with Permission from the American Society for Nutrition

Garlic consumption and cancer prevention: meta-analyses of colorectal and stomach cancers by Aaron T Fleischauer

American Journal of Clinical Nutrition October 1, 2000; 72: 4: 1047-1052.

New Federal Report on Carcinogens Lists Estrogen Therapy, Ultraviolet, Wood Dust

The federal government today published its biennial Report on Carcinogens, adding steroidal estrogens used in estrogen replacement therapy and oral contraceptives to its official list of "known" human carcinogens. This and 15 other new listings bring the total of substances in the report, "known" or "reasonably anticipated" to pose a cancer risk, to 228.

This, the tenth edition of the report, was forwarded to Congress and released to the public today by the Department of Health and Human Services. It was prepared by the National Toxicology Program, an arm of the HHS located at the National Institute of Environmental Health Sciences, one of the National Institutes of Health. The reports are published every two years after lengthy study and scientific reviews by three successive expert panels of government and non-government scientists.

In a statement releasing the report, HHS Secretary Tommy Thompson today thanked "the hundreds of scientists who have contributed to this report through their original research or their careful reviews of these important studies. The public is well served by this dispassionate report that helps all of us ensure that the American public is made aware of potential cancer hazards."

The tenth report newly lists the group of hormones known as steroidal estrogens as "known human carcinogens." A number of the individual steroidal estrogens were already listed as "reasonably anticipated carcinogens" in past editions, but this is the first report to so list all these hormones, as a group. As with all the other medications listed, the Report on Carcinogens does not address or attempt to balance potential benefits of use of these products.

Also newly listed as "known" causes of cancer in humans are broad spectrum ultraviolet radiation, whether generated by the sun or by artificial sources; wood dust created in cutting and shaping wood; nickel compounds and beryllium and its compounds commonly used in industry. Beryllium and beryllium compounds are not new to the list but was previously listed as "reasonably anticipated to be a human carcinogen."

The report is mandated by Congress as a way for the government to help keep the public informed about substances or exposure circumstances that are "known" or are "reasonably anticipated" to cause human cancers. The report also identifies current regulations concerning these listings in an attempt to address how exposures have been reduced.

The report makes a distinction between "known" human carcinogens, where there is sufficient evidence from human studies and "reasonably anticipated" human carcinogens, where there is either limited evidence of carcinogenicity from human studies and/or sufficient evidence of carcinogenicity from experimental animal studies.

The report does not assess the magnitude of the carcinogenic risk, nor does it address any potential benefits of listed substances such as certain pharmaceuticals. Listing in the report does not establish that such substance presents a risk to persons in their daily lives. Such formal risk assessments are the responsibility of Federal, State, and local health regulatory agencies.

Newly listed as known human carcinogens are:

- **Steroidal estrogens**
  These are a group of related hormones that control sex and growth characteristics and are commonly used in *estrogen replacement therapy* to treat symptoms of menopause and in oral contraceptives. The report cites data from human epidemiology studies that show an association between estrogen replacement therapy and a consistent increase in the risk of endometrial cancer (cancer of the endometrial lining of the uterus) and a less consistent increase in the risk of breast cancer.
  As for the other common use for steroidal estrogens, the report says the evidence suggests estrogen-containing oral contraceptives may be associated with an increased risk of breast cancer but may protect against ovarian and endometrial cancers.

- **Broad Spectrum Ultraviolet Radiation (UVR)**
  UVR is produced by the sun as part of solar radiation and by artificial sources such as sun lamps and tanning beds, in medical diagnosis and treatment procedures, and in industry for promoting polymerization reactions. The report cites data indicating a cause-and-effect relationship between this radiation and skin cancer, cancer of the lip and melanoma of the eye. The report goes on to say that skin cancers are observed with increasing duration of exposure and for those who experience sunburn. The individual components of UVR, which includes ultraviolet A, ultraviolet B and ultraviolet C radiation, are listed in the report, not as

"known", but as "reasonably anticipated" human carcinogens—See below.

- **Wood dust**
  Listed as a "known human carcinogen" in this report, wood dust is created when machines and tools cut, shape and finish wood. Wood dust is particularly prevalent in sawmills, furniture manufacture and cabinet making. According to the report, unprotected workers have a higher risk of cancers of the nasal cavities and sinuses.

- **Nickel compounds**
  Used in many industrial applications as catalysts and in batteries, pigments and ceramics, the report newly lists nickel compounds as "known" human carcinogens based on studies of workers showing excess deaths from lung and nasal cancers and on their mechanisms of action.

One group of substances was upgraded from "reasonably anticipated" to "known" human carcinogen:

- **Beryllium and beryllium compounds**
  About 800,000 workers are exposed via inhalation of beryllium dust or dermal contact with products containing beryllium. Workers with the highest potential for exposure include beryllium miners, beryllium alloy makers and fabricators, ceramics workers, missile technicians, nuclear reactor workers, electric and electronic equipment workers, and jewelers. According to data cited in the report, they have higher risks for lung cancer which increase with their exposures and which cannot be explained by tobacco smoking or other occupational exposures.

Twelve substances or groups of substances are newly listed as "reasonably anticipated to be human carcinogens":

- **IQ,** or 2-amino-3-methylimidazo[4,5-f]quinoline, which is formed during direct cooking with high heat of foods such as meats and eggs and also found in cigarette smoke, is listed as "reasonably anticipated to be a human carcinogen" based on long-term animal studies. The report also states there are several published human studies that suggest there is an increased risk for breast and colorectal cancers related to consumption of broiled or fried foods that may contain IQ and/or other similar compounds formed during cooking at high temperatures.

- **2,2-bis-(Bromomethyl)-1,3-propanediol (technical grade),** a flame retardant chemical used to make some polyester resins and rigid polyurethane foam is listed as "reasonably anticipated" based on long-term animal feeding studies.

- **Ultraviolet A, Ultraviolet B and Ultraviolet C Radiation,** are listed as "reasonably anticipated to be human carcinogens" because, according to the report, animal studies show a cause-and-effect relationship between exposure to each of these wavelength groups of broad spectrum ultraviolet radiation (UVR) and skin cancer. The report points out that the data on skin cancer in humans for these different wavelengths of UVR are limited, because it has been impossible to determine if the people in these studies were exposed to "pure" individual components of UVR or, as is more likely the case, to "mixtures" of the different components thus making it impossible to say that the observed skin cancers were due only to one of the "pure" individual components.

- **Chloramphenicol,** An antibiotic with restricted use in the US because it can cause fatal blood disorders, is listed in the report as "reasonably anticipated to be a human carcinogen". The report says the listing is based on limited evidence from human studies that showed an increased cancer risk for the occurrence of leukemia after chloramphenicol therapy.

- **2,3-Dibromo-1-propanol,** a chemical used as an intermediate in the production of flame-retardants, insecticides, and pharmaceuticals, is listed in the report as "reasonably anticipated to be a human carcinogen" based on strong evidence of cancer formation from skin painting study in experimental animals.

- **Dyes metabolized to 3,3'-dimethoxybenzidine** are dyes that have been used to color leather, paper, plastic, rubber and textiles and are listed in the report because they are metabolized to 3,3'-dimethoxybenzidine, which is "reasonably anticipated to be a human carcinogen".

- **Dyes metabolized to 3,3'-demethylbenzidine** are dyes that have been used in printing textiles, in color photography and as biological stains and are listed in the report because these dyes are metabolized to 3,3'-dimethylbenzidine, which is "reasonably anticipated to be a human carcinogen".

- **Methyleugenol,** occurs naturally in oils, herbs and spices and is used in smaller amounts in its natural or synthetic form in flavors, insect attractants, anesthetics and sunscreens. It is listed in the report based on sufficient evidence of cancer formation from oral studies of this chemical in experimental animals.

- **Metallic nickel,** this metal is used mainly in alloys with most exposures by inhalation or skin contact in the workplace. (It should be noted that metallic nickel is not contained in the nickel coin.) It is listed in the report based on sufficient evidence of cancer formation from studies of this chemical in experimental animals.

- **Styrene7,8-oxide,** is used primarily in the production of styrene glycol and its derivatives, as a reactive diluent in epoxy resins, as a treatment for textiles and fibers, and as a chemical intermediate in the manufacture of such materials as perfumes and surface coatings. It is listed in the report based on sufficient evidence of cancer formation from studies of this chemical in experimental animals. (Text corrected July 22, 2003).

- **Vinyl bromide,** which has been used in polymers in making fabrics for clothes and home furnishings, as well as in leather and metal products, drugs and fumigants. It is listed in the report based on sufficient evidence of cancer formation from studies of this chemical in experimental animals.

- **Vinyl fluoride,** which is used in making polyvinyl fluoride and related weather-resistant fluoropolymers. Support for the listing came from inhalation studies in experimental animals. It is listed in the report based on sufficient evidence of cancer formation from studies of this chemical in experimental animals.

Reprinted with permission from the National Institute of Environmental Health Sciences

New Federal Report on Carcinogens Lists Estrogen Therapy, Ultraviolet, Wood Dust (December 11, 2002)

For more data on this topic, have a look at the following website:

National Institute of Environmental Health Sciences:

- **http://www.niehs.nih.gov/oc/news/10thrc.htm**

Fight Cancer by Drinking Green Tea

According to new investigative research, consuming green tea may help thwart the spread of prostate cancer due to the fact that polyphenols found in the tea target molecular pathways that stop the manufacturing and dispersion of tumor cells. They also prevent the growth of tumor-nurturing blood vessels. This particular research study involved using a mouse model for human prostate cancer, indicated the ingestion of green tea polyphenols (GTP) adjusted and decreased levels of the insulin-like growth factor-1 (IGF-1)-driven molecular pathways in prostate tumor cells.

These discoveries gave credit to other studies, which found out that elevated levels of IGF-1 were linked to increased risk of some cancers like:

- Prostate
- Breast
- Lung
- Colon

Experts also found that these GTP inhibited the expression of proteins typically associated with the metastatic spread of cancer cells. This is because the polyphenols prevented the levels of urokinase plasminogen activator as well as cellular molecules linked to the metastasis.

Printed with permission from EurekAlert

Green tea polyphenols thwart prostate cancer development at multiple levels

EurekAlert December 1, 2004

Broccoli & Sprouts Appear to Cut Cancer Risks

A compound found in broccoli and broccoli sprouts appears to be more effective than modern antibiotics against the bacteria which causes peptic ulcers. Moreover, tests in mice show that the compound offers tremendous protection against stomach cancer—the second most common form of cancer in the world. The recent study, led by scientists at Johns Hopkins University, is the latest in a series of studies done in the past 10 years on the cancer-fighting potential of broccoli. (1)

Back in 1992, Johns Hopkins University pharmacology professor Paul Talalay and his colleagues showed that sulforaphane—a substance produced by the body from a compound in broccoli—could trigger the production of phase II enzymes. Phase II enzymes can detoxify cancer-causing chemicals and are among the most potent anti-cancer compounds known to man.

It should be noted that broccoli sprouts have shown to be every bit as beneficial as full grown broccoli.

In another study conducted jointly with US and Chinese researchers (2), it was found that chemicals present in broccoli, cabbage, bok choy, and other cruciferous vegetables may protect against lung cancer. Researchers studied more than 18,000 men. They recorded 259 cases of lung cancer during the study's followup period. The researchers found that the men with detectable amounts of a substance known as "isothiocyanates" in their bodies had a 36% lower risk of developing lung cancer over a 10-year period.

Isothiocyanates are found in broccoli and other so called "cruciferous" vegetables.

Although the chemicals did lower the cancer risk by 36% in this study, it should be noted that smoking alone increases lung cancer risks by as much as 10 times. Smoking is a behavior problem, not some virus that silently comes in and attacks you!

Reprinted with permission from Elsevier.

Isothiocyanates, Glutathione, S-transferase M1 and T1 Polymorphisms, and Lung Cancer Risk: a Prospective Study of men in Shanghai, China by Stephanie J London

1) The Lancet August 26th 2000; 356: 724-729

Reprinted with permission from Proceedings of the National Academy of Sciences (copyright 2002 National Academy of Sciences, USA)

Sulforaphane inhibits extracellular, intracellular, and antibiotic-resistant strains of Helicobacter pylori and prevents benzo[a]pyrene-induced stomach tumors by Jed W. Fahey

2) Proceedings of the National Academy of Sciences May 2002:28; 99(11):7610-7615

Processed Meats May Aid in Developing Colon Cancer

Recent estimates conclude that 3 million to 4 million cases of cancer in the world could be prevented each year through healthy eating and lifestyle alterations. Colon cancer is indeed a great example of this. It is the third most common type of cancer among men and women. Many risk factors increase the chance of developing this illness but high intake of red meat may also be a large contributor. Scientific experts have defined high intake of meat, including beef, veal, pork, sausages and bologna, as three or more ounces a day for men and two or more ounces a day for women.

Experts questioned around 150,000 adults between the ages of 50 and 74 to provide data regarding personal meat consumption in 1982, and again in 1992 or 1993. The results showed that the median intake of red meat was just over 2 ounces a day for men and 1.4 ounces a day for women. Also, the heaviest consumers among men ate 10 times as much red meat than those who ate the least, while the heaviest consumers among women ate 17 times as much.

The Research Showed:

- Individuals who consumed the equivalent of a hamburger a day were about *30 percent to 40 percent more likely* to develop colon cancer than those who ate less than half that amount

- The risk of acquiring colon cancer *increased by 50 percent* with long-term consumption of high amounts of processed meats such as hot dogs

There are two possible theories as to why large amounts of red and processed meats appeared to increase colon cancer risk. They are:

- Cooking meat at high temperatures can lead to the creation of mutagens, which can damage DNA

- High iron content in red meat produces free radicals, which can also damage DNA

Meat Consumption and Risk of Colorectal Cancer by Ann Chao

Journal of the American Medical Association January 12, 2005; 293(2):172-182

Polio Vaccines Implicated in Cancer Development

Quite a few research investigations have found the presence of simian virus 40 (SV40) or protein in human brain tumors and bone cancers, malignant mesothelioma, and non-Hodgkin's lymphoma. However, many of the studies were small or lacking control groups, which made it hard to conclude whether they were reliable. The history of some SV40 infections in humans is associated with the administering of polio vaccines, on a further note.

Referencing conservative estimates, from 1955 to 1963 more than 98 million children and adults in the United States were exposed accidentally to live SV40 because of SV40-contaminated polio vaccines. These polio vaccines were also dispersed to many other countries and different adenovirus vaccines used on some U.S. military personnel from 1961 to 1965 also contained live SV40.

The SV40 virus has been proven to be a powerful oncogenic (cancer producer) deoxyribonucleic acid (DNA) virus and in animal models, the neoplasias induced by SV40 included primary brain cancers, malignant mesotheliomas, bone tumors, and systemic lymphomas.

Polyomavirus SV40 infection prevalence in humans is unknown because there is insufficient data about which individuals received contaminated vaccines and the amount of infectious SV40 in particular lots of vaccine. It is also hard to follow massive groups for years after virus exposure for the development of cancer.

Analysis of molecular biology data shows that polyomavirus SV40 is associated significantly with primary brain and bone cancers, malignant mesothelioma, and non-Hodgkin's lymphoma. Further, SV40 may play a role in the development of the malignancies. One report stated there is moderate strength evidence that SV40 exposure could lead to cancer in humans under natural conditions.

Future studies are needed to determine how SV40 is transmitted and how it interacts with different tissues.

Reprinted with permission from Elsevier

Simian virus 40 in human Cancers by Regis A. Vilchez MD

The American Journal of Medicine June 1, 2003; 114(8):675-684

Tanning Beds Appear to Elevate the Risk of Cancer

Experts warn that the around *1 million* Americans who seek a harmless tan at their local tanning salon *face the same risk of skin cancer as those who are out in the sun excessively.*

Suntan salon exposure *initiates cell damage in the skin,* specifically the type of damage that potentially leads to skin cancer.

Scientific researchers studied 11 males and females with fair skin between the ages of 18 and 50. All subjects were supposedly in good health, and none had gone to the tanning salon within the month prior to the study. Investigators exposed the participants to 10 full-body tanning bed sessions over a 2-week period, using the same types of UV bulbs most commonly found in US tanning salons. The dose of UV exposure was incrementally elevated during subsequent sessions, with a small portion of each participant's skin covered throughout the study and another portion exposed only once at the last session.

The investigators compared skin and blood samples taken from the fully, partially and unexposed skin areas. The experts found that *as a result of the full exposure to the tanning bed's UV bulbs, the participants had alterations in certain parts of their DNA and among certain skin proteins.*

These changes at the molecular level, the team determined, had the possibility to elevate the bed-tanner's long-term risk of developing skin cancer—a risk they stated as being similar to that associated with lying in the sun for prolonged periods.

Many suntan salons prefer to make the claim that their tan is safe, which couldn't be farther from the truth.

The greater the exposures to tanning bed lights, the greater the chances that an individual's skin may not be able to perfectly repair the damage done each time—placing the tanner at an elevated risk of cancer.

Reprinted with permission from the American Academy of Dermatology, Inc. and Elsevier

Tanning salon exposure and molecular alterations by S. Elizabeth Whitmore, MD

Journal of the American Academy of Dermatology May 2001; 44; (8) 775-780

Vitamin D May Shield Against Cancer

Current investigative research suggests that vitamin D may defend against colon cancer by helping to dispose of a toxic acid that propagates the disease. These new findings could lead the way to the progression of therapies that provide the cancer protection of vitamin D without the side effects elicited by ingesting too much of the vitamin.

Right now it is though that we have unlocked the possible mechanism of how vitamin D can be protective of colon cancer. Vitamin D is recognized to shield against cancer of the colon, but exactly how has been unclear. The high-fat "Western" diet is associated with an elevated risk of the illness, although this relationship is contentious.

This current study provides a potential clarification for the protection of vitamin D as well as the elevated risk of a high-fat diet. Experts discovered that vitamin D and a particular type of bile acid called lithocholic acid (LCA) both stimulate the vitamin D receptor in cells. When an individual eats fatty foods, the liver pours bile acids into the intestine, allowing for the body to absorb fatty substances. After performing their task in the intestine, most bile acids are brought back into the liver. LCA does something strange, though. It is not re-circulated into the liver. Instead, an enzyme called CYP3A breaks down LCA in the intestine, he said. If LCA is not detoxified by the enzyme, it drifts into the colon where it can promote cancer.

LCA Is Extremely Toxic

While vitamin D is well established at stopping colon cancer in animals, the expert decided to see whether its receptor had any effect on the detoxification of LCA.

In effect, the vitamin D receptor appears to act as a sensor for elevated levels of LCA. The vitamin D receptor attaches to LCA, catapulting an elevation in the expression of the gene for CYP3A, the acid-neutralizing enzyme. This appears to be the body's way of protecting itself from colon cancer.

If an individual does not get adequate vitamin D, this balance may be disturbed, elevating the risk of colon cancer.

The study also gives a potential explanation of how high-fat diets may raise the risk of colon cancer. Seeing as LCA is released from the liver when an individual consumes fatty food, a high-fat diet that keeps LCA levels high may "overwhelm the system." The body may stop producing enough CYP3A to keep LCA under control.

Reprinted with Permission from Science Magazine (http://www. sciencemag.org/)

Vitamin D Receptor as an Intestinal Bile Acid Sensor by Makoto Makishima

Science May 17, 2002; 296:1313-1316

Antiperspirant Use Appear to Raise Breast Cancer Risks

Using an antiperspirant is one of the more common and dangerous ways individuals are exposed to toxic metals like aluminum. An increasing risk of *breast cancer* is yet another reason to avoid them altogether, according to a study conducted in the UK.

Aluminum salts consist of a quarter of the volume of some antiperspirants, and when they're absorbed into the skin they can begin to imitate and manipulate the estrogen activity that leads to breast cancer. The experts argue that women are especially prone to problems, because they typically use antiperspirants directly after shaving, which allows for easier absorption. There is good news, though. A reduction in your exposure is fairly simple and can be performed by using soap and water to keep your body clean, and getting rid of that antiperspirant.

Additionally, some deodorants aren't as hazardous for your health as are antiperspirants, but I recommend avoiding them as well unless they are 100% organic.

Reprinted with permission from John Wiley and Sons Limited.

Metalloestrogens: an emerging class of inorganic xenoestrogens with potential to add to the oestrogenic burden of the human breast by P. D. Darbre

Journal of Applied Toxicology (May/June 2006) Volume 26, Issue 3, pg 191-197

Birth Control Pills May Raise Cancer Risk

Elder generation birth-control pills may have considerably elevated breast cancer risk among women with a family history of the disease. Scientific experts studied 426 families and found that *oral contraceptive use tripled breast cancer risk* among women with sisters or mothers who were stricken with the illness.

An elevated cancer risk was isolated to women who used birth control pills before 1975.

Now oral contraceptives have evolved to include lower doses of estrogen and progestin, which may make them safer in terms of breast cancer, scientific experts suggest, although this will likely not be definitively known for years to come.

The breast cancer association was at its peak among women with five or more cases of breast or ovarian cancer in their families. In these particular women, birth control pill intake was linked to an 11-fold elevation in breast cancer risk.

Reprinted with permission from the American Medical Association. All rights reserved.

Risk of Breast Cancer With Oral Contraceptive Use in Women With a Family History of Breast Cancer by Dawn M. Grabrick

Oral Contraceptives and Breast Cancer: A Note of Caution for High-Risk Women by Wylie Burke

The Journal of the American Medical Association October 11, 2000; 284: (14): 1791-1798, 1837-1838

Raspberries May Help Prevent Throat Cancer

Experts suggest black raspberries might hold compounds that thwart esophageal cancer and keep precancerous growths from becoming malignant. In referencing the study, *rats injected with a cancer-causing compound were less likely to develop cancer of the esophagus when black raspberries comprised 5% to 10% of their daily diet.* The results add to an ever expanding body of evidence associating a lower cancer risk with berry consumption.

Raspberries consist of many vitamins, minerals, plant constituents and antioxidants referred to as anthocyanins that might defend against cancer. It is uncertain how these compounds thwart off cancer but experts recommend that individuals include a serving of fresh or frozen berries in their daily diet.

The researchers in this study injected rats with NMBA, a toxin that has an association with esophageal cancer. Some rats had a diet comprised of 5% to 10% black raspberries before and/or after receiving injections, while other rats were fed diets that excluded raspberries. It was found that rats which consumed the highest quantity of black raspberries both 2 weeks before and up to 30 weeks after NMBA injections had 49% less tumors than rats whose diets excluded black raspberries, scientific experts stated. In addition, tumors that had developed in rats fed raspberries only after getting the injections were reported to go down in size after 15 weeks. After 25 weeks, rats fed diets of 5% to 10% black raspberries watched the number of esophageal tumors drop by 43% to 62%. A diet consisting of 5% black raspberries was more effective than a diet consisting of 10% black raspberries.

Cancer of the esophagus is the fifth leading cause of cancer death in the entire world, according to the report. Only 8% to 12% of people will live 5 years after being diagnosed with the illness.

Reprinted with permission from the American Association of Cancer Research

Chemoprevention of Esophageal Tumorigenesis by Dietary Administration of Lyophilized Black Raspberries by Laura A. Kresty

Cancer Research August 2001; 61: 6112-6119

Applying Sunscreen May Not Prevent Melanoma

Experts are uncertain whether sunscreen prevents melanoma from developing, the most deadly type of skin cancer that is responsible for greater than 75 percent of skin cancer fatalities. They imply that sunscreen may prevent sunburn, but may fail to defend against cancer. Sunscreens are manufactured to absorb energy from ultraviolet light, but the energy may be transferred to the DNA in skin cells, which could wreak havoc.

Previous research has even found an association with melanoma and sunscreen use, though experts suggest this might only show that individuals who are easily sunburned, who are more likely to acquire melanoma, are also more likely to use sunscreen.

Scientific experts still advise using sunscreen as it does shield against basal cell carcinoma (the most frequent type of skin cancer that is usually easy to treat), and sunburn, and it slows the wrinkling of aging skin.

Reprinted with permission from The Baltimore Sun

Sunscreen May let in Deadly Rays by Scott Shane

The Baltimore Sun July 14, 2003

Statin Drugs NOT Effective in Preventing Cancer

Statin drugs, a class of accepted cholesterol-lowering drugs, are not protective against cancer, despite the preliminary indications of some older research studies. The first study looked at total cancer risk, and the other focused solely on colon cancer. In the two studies, patients consuming statin drugs proved just as likely to develop cancer as anyone else.

Experts examining the research confirmed that those wanting to avoid cancer should not rely on experimental therapies. For those concerned about colon cancer, colonoscopies allow polyps to be removed before they turn malignant, reducing the cancer risk by 80 percent to 90 percent.

The expert behind one of the studies recommended following verified steps to prevent cancer, such as stopping smoking, exercising, and controlling your weight.

Reprinted with permission from the American Medical Association. All rights reserved.

Statins and Cancer Risk: A Meta-analysis by Krista M. Dale

Journal of the American Medical Association January 4, 2006; 295(1): 74-80

Prostate Cancer Slowed Down by Pomegranate Extract

New evidence has surfaced showing pomegranate juice may help fight prostate cancer. Pomegranates are high in anti-oxidant and anti-inflammatory content, and have proven effective on tumors in mouse skin.

Scientific experts first analyzed various doses of pomegranate extract on human prostate cancer cells cultured in the lab. The greater the dose of pomegranate extract, the more of these cells died. After that, they examined mice which had been injected with prostate cancer cells. Mice who received the equivalent of the amount of pomegranate juice a human might be willing to ingest daily showed a dramatic slowing of the progression of their cancer, as compared to mice which were given lesser dosages or only water. Now, the next step in analyzing pomegranates for cancer treatment and prevention will be tests used on humans.

Cancer of the prostate is the second leading cause of cancer death in American men. Greater than 230,000 new cases of prostate cancer are anticipated to be diagnosed this year alone in the United States.

Printed with permission from EurekAlert

Can pomegranates prevent prostate cancer? A new study offers promise

EurekAlert University of Wisconsin-Madison September 26, 2005

Breast Cancer Risk May Increase by 50% from Consistent Aspirin and Ibuprofen Use

A recent study furthers the concern that taking aspirin or ibuprofen may significantly increase a woman's chance of developing to breast cancer. These new discoveries merely stress concerns about the possible toxicities amounting from long-term regular consumption of nonsteroidal anti-inflammatory drugs (NSAIDs).

Scientific experts examined information on around 114,000 females (ages 22-85) who participated in the California Teachers Study. The females did not have breast cancer when they enrolled in the research study ten years ago. During that time, the women informed the experts how often and how long they had ingested aspirin and ibuprofen.

Throughout the follow-up period, roughly 2,400 of the women were diagnosed with breast cancer of known receptor status. As the scientific experts broke their findings down by pain reliever or type of breast cancer, the findings were:

- Taking ibuprofen every day for at least five years increased a woman's chance of developing breast cancer by 50 percent, compared to women who did not regularly take the drug.

- Daily use of aspirin for five years or more caused a woman's risk of ER/PR-negative breast cancer (not sensitive to estrogen or progesterone) to spike by 80 percent, compared to non-regular aspirin users.

Printed with permission from EurekAlert

Study examines NSAID use and breast cancer risk

EurekAlert May 30, 2005

Breast Cancer Risk Raises with PCB Exposure

One new study's discoveries confirm that elevated levels of specific polychlorinated biphenyls (PCB's) may be connected to breast cancer. These unrelenting environmental contaminants can build up in the body of women with age and are comparable in structure to dioxin which may be a risk factor for breast cancer. Scientific experts also emphasize the importance of additional research on the potential connection between environmental contaminants that can mimic or change hormone metabolism and the risk of breast cancer.

PCBs are classified as a group of chemicals with various industrial and commercial applications. PCBs were barred in the US and Canada two decades ago because of worries about the health effects of the chemicals. The chemicals still remain in the environment and are present in the food chain, predominantly in fatty foods.

In the last ten years, numerous studies have presented the potential connection between exposure to PCBs and an elevated risk of breast cancer. Many studies did not find a link between increased levels of the chemicals and breast cancer, but much of the research examined at overall levels of PCBs, not individual chemicals. Experts reviewed the link between breast cancer risk and 14 individual PCBs in 314 women with breast cancer and a "control" group of 523 healthy women.

Levels of two PCBs (PCB 118 and PCB 156) were associated with a *60% to 80% greater risk of breast cancer,* the experts found. This connection was more pronounced in premenopausal females. This investigative research also discovered that females with increased levels of a combination of three PCBs that imitate the cancer-causing chemical dioxin (PCBs 105, 118 and 156) were about two times as likely to have breast cancer. This risk was also elevated in premenopausal females.

Findings may suggest a link between dioxin-like constituents and breast cancer risk. This is the second largest study to indicate a relationship between PCBs and breast cancer.

Reprinted with permission from Oxford University Press

Plasma Concentrations of Polychlorinated Biphenyls and the Risk of Breast Cancer: A Congener-specific Analysis by Alain Demers

American Journal of Epidemiology April 1, 2002; 155: (7): 629-635

Exercise Shown to Decrease Ovarian Cancer Risk

A new study confirms, females who stay highly active throughout life are less apt to develop ovarian cancer.

- Scientific experts analyzed more than 2,100 women and discovered that *those who exercised more than 6 hours per week were 27% less likely to develop ovarian cancer than women who exercised less than 1 hour each week.*

- High activity levels protected women of all ages. However, less than one quarter of the women exercised at that level.

- Older studies have linked exercise to a decreased risk of breast cancer

- Highly active females in this study regularly showed decreased ovarian cancer risk across all age groups, from age 20 to 69.

Scientific experts hypothesize that exercise may cut cancer risk by:

- Preventing obesity
- Hormonal Effects of exercise
- Exercise could be simply be a marker for a generally healthful lifestyle.

Reprinted with permission from Lippincott, Williams, & Wilkins

Physical Activity and Reduced Risk of Ovarian Cancer by Carrie M. Cottreau

Obstetrics and Gynecology October 2000; 96: (4): 609-14

Cancer Risk Elevated by Farmed Salmon Intake

Investigative experts from the United States expressed concern that farm-raised salmon have significantly elevated levels of toxins, such as PCBs, than wild salmon. The most tainted fish were from Scotland and the Faroe Islands, and experts observed that concentrations of all contaminants were drastically higher among salmon farm-raised in Europe, in contrast to those farm-raised in North and South America.

Experts looked at farm-raised Atlantic salmon and investigated the levels of 14 toxins that were likely to cause cancer in people. Experts discovered significantly heightened levels of 13 toxins in contrast to wild pacific salmon. The researchers performed morel studies on four contaminants that are proven to be dangerous to human health: PCBs, dioxins, toxaphene and dieldrin. They found concentrations of these chemicals were time and again greater in farmed salmon than fish from the wild.

Scientists are now suggesting people consume no more than two ounces of Scottish farmed salmon each month. They also suggest that people may want to stay away from Atlantic salmon, which is virtually all farm raised, and seek out Alaskan king salmon or other wild salmon instead until new guidelines are developed.

After the research, the United States denied entry to salmon from Scottish fish farms after U.S. after tests showed the shipments were "unfit for human consumption." The Observer stated, "Last year 15 shipments of smoked salmon were turned away because they were contaminated with listeria. A further nine salmon shipments from Scotland were classified as *unsanitary*. According to the FDA, they *may have become contaminated with filth* and *may have been rendered injurious to health*. Three more salmon shipments were officially defined as filthy."

Reprinted with Permission from Science Magazine (http://www. sciencemag.org/)

Global Assessment of Organic Contaminants in Farmed Salmon by Ronald A. Hites

Science January 9, 2004; 303 (5655):226-229

Kelp May Decrease Breast Cancer Risk

Kelp seaweed may be promising as a new cancer-fighting food, particularly to treat breast cancer, in reference to recent research. Experts found a diet including kelp seaweed, a little studied nutrient, decreased levels of the powerful sex hormone estradiol in rats, elevating hopes it may drop the risk of estrogen-dependent illnesses. The type of kelp used in this study (bladderwrack seaweed (Fucus vesiculosus)) is closely associated to wakame and kombu, the brown seaweeds most frequently eaten in Japan and the chief form of kelp sold in this country.

Studies before have suggested Japanese females have longer menstrual cycles and lower serum estradiol levels than their Western counterparts, which investigators state may add to their lower rates of breast, endometrial and ovarian cancers. Experts arbitrarily divided 24 female rats into three groups that got either a high (70 milligrams) or low dose (35 milligrams) of dried, powdered kelp for four weeks or none at all. After using daily vaginal swabs to monitor the rats' menstrual cycles, scientists discovered their estrous cycles elevated from an average of 4.3 to 5.4 days for the low dose kelp group, and to 5.9 days for the high dose kelp group.

In total, dietary kelp culminated in a 37 percent elevation in the length of a rat's estrous cycle. Human studies have associated longer menstrual cycles to a decreased risk of breast, ovarian and endometrial cancers. By having less periods, experts say, not as much time is spent overall in phases where hormone levels and breast and endometrial cell proliferation are at their greatest.

Reprinted with permission from the American Society for Nutrition

Brown Kelp Modulates Endocrine Hormones in Female Sprague-Dawley Rats and in Human Luteinized Granulosa Cells by Christine F. Skibola

Journal of Nutrition 135: 2: 296-300, February 2005

The Doors of Perception: Why Americans Will Believe Almost Anything

by Dr. Tim O'Shea

www.mercola.com

We are the most conditioned, programmed beings the world has ever known. Not only are our thoughts and attitudes continually being shaped and molded; our very awareness of the whole design seems like it is being subtly and inexorably erased.

The doors of our perception are carefully and precisely regulated. Who cares, right?

It is an exhausting and endless task to keep explaining to people how most issues of conventional wisdom are scientifically implanted in the public consciousness by a thousand media clips per day. In an effort to save time, I would like to provide just a little background on the handling of information in this country.

Once the basic principles are illustrated about how our current system of media control arose historically, the reader might be more apt to question any given story in today's news.

If everybody believes something, it's probably wrong. We call that Conventional Wisdom.

In America, conventional wisdom that has mass acceptance is usually contrived: somebody paid for it. Examples:

- Pharmaceuticals restore health
- Vaccination brings immunity
- The cure for cancer is just around the corner
- When a child is sick, he needs immediate antibiotics
- When a child has a fever he needs Tylenol
- Hospitals are safe and clean.
- America has the best health care in the world.

- And many many more

This is a list of illusions that have cost billions and billions to conjure up. Did you ever wonder why you never see the President speaking publicly unless he is reading? Or why most people in this country think generally the same about most of the above issues?

How This Set-Up Got Started

In *Trust Us We're Experts*, Stauber and Rampton pull together some compelling data describing the science of creating public opinion in America.

They trace modern public influence back to the early part of the last century, highlighting the work of guys like Edward L. Bernays, the Father of Spin. From his own amazing chronicle Propaganda, we learn how Edward L. Bernays took the ideas of his famous uncle Sigmund Freud himself, and applied them to the emerging science of mass persuasion.

The only difference was that instead of using these principles to uncover hidden themes in the human unconscious, the way Freudian psychology does, Bernays used these same ideas to mask agendas and to create illusions that deceive and misrepresent, for marketing purposes.

The Father Of Spin

Bernays dominated the PR industry until the 1940s, and was *a significant force* for another 40 years after that. (Tye) During all that time, Bernays took on hundreds of diverse assignments to *create a public perception about some idea or product*. A few examples:

As a neophyte with the Committee on Public Information, one of Bernays' first assignments was to help sell the First World War to the American public with the idea to "Make the World Safe for Democracy." (Ewen)

A few years later, Bernays set up a stunt to popularize the notion of women smoking cigarettes. In organizing the 1929 Easter Parade in New York City, Bernays showed himself as *a force to be reckoned with*.

He organized the Torches of Liberty Brigade in which suffragettes marched in the parade smoking cigarettes as a mark of women's liberation. Such publicity followed from that one event that from then on women have felt secure about destroying their own lungs in public, the same way that men have always done.

Bernays popularized the idea of bacon for breakfast.

Not one to turn down a challenge, he set up the advertising format along with the AMA that lasted for nearly 50 years proving that cigarettes are beneficial to health. Just look at ads in issues of Life or Time from the 40s and 50s.

Smoke And Mirrors

Bernay's job was to *reframe an issue*; to create a desired image that would put a particular product or concept in a desirable light. Bernays described the public as a 'herd that needed to be led.' And this herdlike thinking makes people "susceptible to leadership."

Bernays never deviated from his fundamental axiom to "control the masses without their knowing it." The best PR happens with the people unaware that they are being manipulated.

Stauber describes Bernays' rationale like this:

"the scientific manipulation of public opinion was necessary to overcome chaos and conflict in a democratic society." Trust Us p 42

These early mass persuaders postured themselves as performing a moral service for humanity in general—democracy was too good for people; they *needed to be told what to think,* because they were incapable of rational thought by themselves. Here's a paragraph from Bernays' Propaganda:

"Those who manipulate the unseen mechanism of society constitute an invisible government which is the true ruling power of our country. We are governed, our minds molded, our tastes formed, our ideas suggested largely by men we have never heard of.

This is a logical result of the way in which our democratic society is organized. Vast numbers of human beings must cooperate in this manner if they are to live together as a smoothly functioning society.

In almost every act of our lives whether in the sphere of politics or business in our social conduct or our ethical thinking, we are dominated by the relatively small number of persons who understand the mental processes and social patterns of the masses. It is they who pull the wires that control the public mind."

Here Comes The Money

Once the possibilities of applying Freudian psychology to mass media were glimpsed, Bernays soon had more corporate clients than he could handle. Global corporations fell all over themselves courting the new Image Makers. There were dozens of goods and services and ideas to be *sold to a susceptible public.* Over the years, these players have had the money to make their images happen. A few examples:

Philip Morris	Pfizer	Union Carbide
Allstate	Monsanto	Eli Lilly
tobacco industry	Ciba Geigy	lead industry
Coors	DuPont	Chlorox
Shell Oil	Standard Oil	Procter & Gamble
Boeing	General Motors	Dow Chemical
General Mills	Goodyear	

The Players

Though world-famous within the PR industry, the companies have names we don't know, and for good reason.

The best PR goes unnoticed.

For decades they have created the opinions that most of us were raised with, on virtually any issue which has the remotest commercial value, including:

pharmaceutical drugs	vaccines
medicine as a profession	alternative medicine
fluoridation of city water	chlorine
household cleaning products	tobacco
dioxin	global warming
leaded gasoline	cancer research and treatment

pollution of the oceans	forests and lumber
images of celebrities, including damage control	crisis and disaster management
genetically modified foods	aspartame
food additives; processed foods	dental amalgams

Lesson #1

Bernays learned early on that the most effective way to create credibility for a product or an image was by "*independent third-party*" endorsement.

For example, if General Motors were to come out and say that global warming is a hoax thought up by some liberal tree-huggers, people would suspect GM's motives, since GM's fortune is made by selling automobiles.

If however some independent research institute with a very credible sounding name like the Global Climate Coalition comes out with a scientific report that says global warming is really a fiction, people begin to get confused and to have doubts about the original issue.

So that's exactly what Bernays did. With a policy inspired by genius, he set up "more institutes and foundations than Rockefeller and Carnegie combined." (Stauber p 45)

Quietly financed by the industries whose products were being evaluated, these "independent" research agencies would churn out "scientific" studies and press materials that could *create any image their handlers wanted.* Such front groups are given high-sounding names like:

Temperature Research Foundation	Manhattan Institute
International Food Information Council	Center for Produce Quality
Consumer Alert	Tobacco Institute Research Council
The Advancement of Sound Science Coalition	Cato Institute
Air Hygiene Foundation	American Council on Science and Health
Industrial Health Federation	Global Climate Coalition
International Food Information Council	Alliance for Better Foods

Sound pretty legit, don't they?

Canned News Releases

As Stauber explains, these organizations and hundreds of others like them are front groups whose sole mission is to advance the image of the global corporations who fund them, like those listed on page 2 above.

This is accomplished in part by an endless stream of 'press releases' announcing "breakthrough" research to every radio station and newspaper in the country. (Robbins) Many of these canned reports read like straight news, and indeed are purposely molded in the news format.

This saves journalists the trouble of researching the subjects on their own, especially on topics about which they know very little. Entire sections of the release or in the case of video news releases, the whole thing can be just lifted intact, with no editing, given the byline of the reporter or newspaper or TV station—and voilá! Instant news—copy and paste. Written by corporate PR firms.

Does this really happen? Every single day since the 1920s when the idea of the News Release was first invented by Ivy Lee. (Stauber, p 22) Sometimes as many as half the stories appearing in an issue of the Wall St. Journal are based solely on such PR press releases. (22)

These types of stories are *mixed right in with legitimately researched stories.* Unless you have done the research yourself, you won't be able to tell the difference.

The Language Of Spin

As 1920s spin pioneers like Ivy Lee and Edward Bernays gained more experience, they began to formulate *rules and guidelines for creating public opinion.* They learned quickly that mob psychology must focus on emotion, not facts. Since the mob is incapable of rational thought, motivation must be based not on logic but on presentation. Here are some of the axioms of the new science of PR:

- technology is a religion unto itself
- if people are incapable of rational thought, real democracy is dangerous
- important decisions should be left to experts
- when reframing issues, stay away from substance; create images

- never state a clearly demonstrable lie

Words are very carefully chosen for their emotional impact. Here's an example. A front group called the International Food Information Council handles the public's natural aversion to genetically modified foods.

Trigger words are repeated all through the text. Now in the case of GM foods, the public is instinctively afraid of these experimental new creations which have suddenly popped up on our grocery shelves which are said to have DNA alterations. The IFIC wants to reassure the public of the safety of GM foods, so it avoids words like:

Frankenfoods	Hitler	biotech
chemical	DNA	experiments
manipulate	money	safety
scientists	radiation	roulette
gene-splicing	gene gun	random

Instead, good PR for GM foods contains words like:

hybrids	natural order	beauty
choice	bounty	cross-breeding
diversity	earth	farmer
organic	wholesome	

It's basic Freudian/Tony Robbins *word association*. The fact that GM foods are not hybrids that have been subjected to the slow and careful scientific methods of real crossbreeding doesn't really matter. This is pseudoscience, not science. Form is everything and substance just a passing myth. (Trevanian)

Who do you think funds the International Food Information Council? Take a wild guess. Right—Monsanto, DuPont, Frito-Lay, Coca Cola, Nutrasweet—those in a position to make fortunes from GM foods. (Stauber p 20)

Characteristics Of Good Propaganda

As the science of mass control evolved, PR firms developed further guidelines for effective copy. Here are some of the gems:

- dehumanize the attacked party by labeling and name calling
- speak in glittering generalities using emotionally positive words
- when covering something up, don't use plain English; stall for time; distract
- get endorsements from celebrities, churches, sports figures, street people—anyone who has no expertise in the subject at hand
- the 'plain folks' ruse: us billionaires are just like you
- when minimizing outrage, don't say anything memorable, point out the benefits of what just happened, and avoid moral issues

Keep this list. Start watching for these techniques. Not hard to find—look at today's paper or tonight's TV news. See what they're doing; these guys are good!

Science For Hire

PR firms have become very sophisticated in the preparation of news releases. They have learned how to attach the names of famous scientists to research that those scientists have not even looked at. (Stauber, p 201)

This is a common occurrence. In this way the editors of newspapers and TV news shows are often not even aware that an individual release is a total PR fabrication. Or at least they have "deniability," right?

Stauber tells the amazing story of how leaded gas came into the picture. In 1922, General Motors discovered that adding lead to gasoline gave cars more horsepower.

When there was some concern about safety, GM paid the Bureau of Mines to do some fake "testing" and publish spurious research that 'proved' that inhalation of lead was harmless. Enter Charles Kettering.

Founder of the world famous Sloan-Kettering Memorial Institute for medical research, Charles Kettering also happened to be an executive with General Motors.

By some strange coincidence, we soon have the Sloan Kettering institute issuing reports stating that lead occurs naturally in the body and that the body has a way of eliminating low level exposure.

Through its association with The Industrial Hygiene Foundation and PR giant Hill & Knowlton, Sloane Kettering opposed all anti-lead research for years. (Stauber p 92). Without organized scientific opposition, for the next *60 years* more and more gasoline became leaded, until by the 1970s, 90% of our gasoline was leaded.

Finally it became *too obvious to hide* that lead was a major carcinogen, and leaded gas was phased out in the late 1980s. But during those 60 years, it is estimated that some 30 million tons of lead were released in vapor form onto American streets and highways. 30 million tons.

That is PR, my friends.

Junk Science

In 1993 a guy named Peter Huber wrote a new book and coined a new term. The book was Galileo's Revenge and the term was junk science. Huber's shallow thesis was that real science supports technology, industry, and progress.

Anything else was suddenly junk science. Not surprisingly, Stauber explains how Huber's book was supported by the industry-backed Manhattan Institute.

Huber's book was generally dismissed not only because it was so poorly written, but because it failed to realize one fact: true scientific research begins with no conclusions. Real scientists are seeking the truth because *they do not yet know what the truth is.*

True scientific method goes like this:

1. Form a hypothesis
2. Make predictions for that hypothesis
3. Test the predictions
4. Reject or revise the hypothesis based on the research findings

Boston University scientist Dr. David Ozonoff explains that ideas in science are themselves like "living organisms that must be nourished, supported, and cultivated with resources for making them *grow and flourish.*" (Stauber p 205)

Great ideas that don't get this financial support because the commercial angles are not immediately obvious—these ideas wither and die.

Another way you can often distinguish real science from phony is that real science points out flaws in its own research. Phony science pretends there were no flaws.

The Real Junk Science

Contrast this with modern PR and its constant pretensions to sound science. Corporate sponsored research, whether it's in the area of drugs, GM foods, or chemistry begins with predetermined conclusions.

It is the job of the scientists then to prove that these conclusions are true, because of the economic upside that proof will bring to the industries paying for that research. This invidious approach to science has shifted the entire focus of research in America during the past 50 years, as any true scientist is likely to admit.

Stauber documents the increasing amount of corporate sponsorship of university research. (206) This has nothing to do with the pursuit of knowledge. Scientists lament that research has become just another commodity, something bought and sold. (Crossen)

The Two Main Targets Of "Sound Science"

It is shocking when Stauber shows how the vast majority of corporate PR today opposes any research that seeks to protect

- public health
- the environment

It's a funny thing that most of the time when we see the phrase "junk science," it is in a context of defending something that may threaten either the environment or our health.

This makes sense when one realizes that money changes hands only by selling the illusion of health and the illusion of environmental protection. *True public health and real preservation* of the earth's environment have very low market value.

Stauber thinks it ironic that industry's self-proclaimed debunkers of junk science are usually non-scientists themselves. (255) Here again they can do this because the issue is not science, but the creation of images.

The Language Of Attack

When PR firms attack legitimate environmental groups and alternative medicine people, they again use special words which will carry an emotional punch:

outraged sound science	junk science sensible	scaremongering responsible
phobia hoax	alarmist hysteria	

The next time you are reading a newspaper article about an environmental or health issue, note how the author shows bias by using the above terms. This is the result of very *specialized training.*

Another standard PR tactic is to *use the rhetoric of the environmentalists themselves to defend a dangerous and untested product that poses an actual threat* to the environment. This we see constantly in the PR smokescreen that surrounds genetically modified foods.

They talk about how GM foods are necessary to grow more food and to end world hunger, when the reality is that GM foods actually have lower yields per acre than natural crops. (Stauber p 173)

The grand design sort of comes into focus once you realize that almost all GM foods have been created by the sellers of herbicides and pesticides so that those plants can withstand greater amounts of herbicides and pesticides. (The Magic Bean)

Kill Your TV?

Hope this chapter has given you a hint to start reading newspaper and magazine articles a little differently, and perhaps start watching TV news shows with a slightly different attitude than you had before.

Always ask, what are they selling here, and who's selling it? And if you actually follow up on Stauber & Rampton's book and check out some of the other resources below, you might even glimpse the possibility of advancing your life one quantum simply by *ceasing to subject your brain to mass media.*

That's right—no more newspapers, no more TV news, no more Time magazine or Newsweek. You could actually do that. Just think what you could do with the extra time alone.

Really feel like you need to "relax" or find out "what's going on in the world" for a few hours every day? Think about the news of the past couple of years for a minute.

Do you really suppose the major stories that have dominated headlines and TV news have been "what is going on in the world?" Do you actually think there's been nothing going on besides the contrived tech slump, the contrived power shortages, the re-filtered accounts of foreign violence and disaster, and all the other non-stories that the puppeteers dangle before us every day?

What about when they get a big one, like with OJ or Monica Lewinsky or the Oklahoma city bombing? Do we really need to know all that detail, day after day? Do we have *any way of verifying all that detail,* even if we wanted to? What is the purpose of news?

To inform the public? Hardly. The sole purpose of news is to *keep the public in a state of fear and uncertainty* so that they'll watch again tomorrow and be subjected to the same advertising.

Oversimplification? Of course. That's the mark of mass media mastery—simplicity. The invisible hand. Like Edward Bernays said, the people must be controlled without them knowing it.

Consider this: what was really going on in the world all that time they were distracting us with all that stupid vexatious daily smokescreen? Fear and uncertainty—that's what keeps people coming back for more.

If this seems like a radical outlook, let's take it one step further:

What would you lose from your life if you stopped watching TV and stopped reading newspapers altogether?

Would your life really suffer any financial, moral, intellectual or academic loss from such a decision?

Do you really need to have your family continually absorbing the illiterate, amoral, phony, uncultivated, desperately brainless values of the people featured in the average nightly TV program? Are these fake, programmed robots "normal"?

Do you need to have your life values constantly spoon-fed to you?

Are those shows really amusing, or just a necessary distraction to keep you from looking at reality, or trying to figure things out yourself by doing a little independent reading?

Name one example of how your life is improved by watching TV news and reading the evening paper.

What measurable gain is there for you?

Planet of the Apes?

There's no question that as a nation, *we're getting dumber year by year.* Look at the presidents we've been choosing lately. Ever notice the blatant grammar mistakes so ubiquitous in today's advertising and billboards?

Literacy is marginal in most American secondary schools. Three fourths of California high school seniors can't read well enough to pass their exit exams. (SJ Mercury 20 Jul 01)

If you think other parts of the country are smarter, try this one: hand any high school senior a book by Dumas or Jane Austen, and ask them to open to any random page and just read one paragraph out loud. Go ahead, do it. *SAT scales are arbitrarily shifted lower* and lower to disguise how dumb kids are getting year by year.

At least 10% have documented "learning disabilities," which are reinforced and rewarded by special treatment and special drugs. Ever hear of anyone failing a grade any more?

Or observe the intellectual level of the average movie which these days may only last one or two weeks in the theatres, especially if it has insufficient explosions, chase scenes, silicone, fake martial arts, and cretinesque dialogue.

Radio? Consider the low mental qualifications of the falsely animated corporate simians they hire as DJs—they're only allowed to have 50 thoughts, which they just repeat at random.

And at what point did popular music cease to require the study of any musical instrument or theory whatsoever, not to mention lyric? Perhaps we just don't understand this emerging art form, right? The Darwinism of MTV—apes descended from man.

Ever notice how most articles in any of the glossy magazines sound like they were all written by the same guy? And this guy just graduated from junior college? And yet he has all the correct opinions on social issues, no original ideas, and that shallow, smug, homogenized corporate omniscience, which enables him to assure us that everything is going to be fine...

All this is great news for the PR industry—makes their job that much easier. Not only are very few paying attention to the process of conditioning; *fewer are capable of understanding it even if somebody explained it to them.*

Tea In the Cafeteria

Let's say you're in a crowded cafeteria, and you buy a cup of tea. And as you're about to sit down you see your friend way across the room. So you put the tea down and walk across the room and talk to your friend for a few minutes.

Now, coming back to your tea, are you just going to pick it up and drink it? Remember, this is a crowded place and you've just left your tea unattended for several minutes. You've given anybody in that room access to your tea.

Why should your mind be any different? Turning on the TV, or uncritically absorbing mass publications every day—these activities allow access to our minds by "just anyone"—anyone who has an agenda, anyone with the resources to create a public image via popular media.

As we've seen above, *just because we read something or see something on TV doesn't mean it's true* or worth knowing. So the idea here is, like the tea, the mind is also worth guarding, worth limiting access to it.

This is the only life we get. Time is our total capital. Why waste it allowing our potential, our personality, our values to be shaped, crafted, and limited according to the whims of the mass panderers?

There are many important issues that are crucial to our physical, mental, and spiritual well-being. If it's an issue where money is involved, objective data won't be so easy to obtain. Remember, if everybody knows something, that image has been bought and paid for.

Real knowledge takes a little effort, a little excavation down at least one level below what "everybody knows."

Reprinted with Permission from mercola.com

http://www.mercola.com/2001/aug/15/perception.htm

References

Stauber & Rampton, "Trust Us, We're Experts", Tarcher/Putnam 2001

Ewen, Stuart PR!: A Social History of Spin 1996 ISBN: 0-465-06168-0 Published by Basic Books, A Division of Harper Collins

Tye, Larry The Father of Spin: Edward L. Bernays and the Birth of Public Relations Crown Publishers, Inc. 2001

King, R Medical journals rarely disclose researchers' ties Wall St. Journal, 2 Feb 99.

Engler, R et al. Misrepresentation and Responsibility in Medical Research New England Journal of Medicine v 317 p 1383 26 Nov 1987

Black, D PhD Health At the Crossroads Tapestry 1988. revanian Shibumi 1983.

Crossen, C Tainted Truth: The Manipulation of Fact in America 1996.

Robbins, J Reclaiming Our Health Kramer 1996.

O'Shea T The Magic Bean 2000.

Inhibitory effect of conjugated dienoic derivatives of linoleic acid and beta-carotene on the in vitro growth of human cancer cells CANCER LETT. (Ireland), 1992, 63/2 (125-133)

Inhibition of Listeria monocytogenes by fatty acids and monoglycerides APPL. ENVIRON. MICROBIOL. (USA), 1992, 58/2 (624-629)

Expert Deception: PR Media Industry Exposed

by Tate Hausman

Think about how many times you've heard an evening news anchor spit out some variation on the phrase, "According to experts...." It's such a common device that most of us hardly hear it anymore. But we do hear the "expert"—the professor or doctor or watchdog group—tell us whom to vote for, what to eat, when to buy stock. And, most of the time, we trust them. Now ask yourself, how many times has that news anchor revealed who those experts are, where they get their funding, and what constitutes their political agenda? If you answered never, you'd be close.

That's the driving complaint behind *Trust Us, We're Experts*, a new book co-authored by John Stauber and Sheldon Rampton of the Center for Media and Democracy. Unlike many so-called "experts," the Center's agenda is quite overt—to expose the shenanigans of the public relations industry, which pays, influences and even invents a startling number of those experts.

The third book co-authored by Stauber and Rampton, *Trust Us* hit bookstore shelves in January. We caught up with John Stauber, who is currently on a nationwide publicity tour, to ask him a few questions about the book, the PR industry and the egregious manipulation of facts for corporate profit.

Tate Hausman: What was the most surprising or disturbing manipulation of public opinion you reveal in your book?

John Stauber: The most disturbing aspect is not a particular example, but rather the fact that the news media regularly fails to investigate so-called "independent experts" associated with industry front groups. They all have friendly-sounding names like "Consumer Alert" and "The Advancement of Sound Science Coalition," but they fail to reveal their corporate funding and their propaganda agenda, which is to smear legitimate heath and community safety concerns as "junk-science fear-mongering."

The news media frequently uses the term "junk science" to smear environmental health advocates. The PR industry has spent more than a decade and many millions of dollars funding and creating industry front groups which wrap them in the flag of "sound science." In reality, their "sound science" is progress as defined by the tobacco industry, the drug industry, the chemical industry, the genetic engineering industry, the petroleum industry and so on.

Hausman: Have you taken heat from the PR industry about this or any of your previous work?

Stauber: We are occasionally attacked in print by PR professionals, but the more prevalent attitude shared with us off the record is to compliment our work, and tell us that we have an accurate portrayal of the business of propaganda, but that in fact all that goes on in the PR world is even worse that we can imagine. I always respond by telling the PR worker that they should write their own book, bare their soul and educate the public about their years of propaganda for firms like Edelman, Burson-Marsteller, Ketchum and the rest. But that usually short-circuits the conversation.

Hausman: Is the public becoming more aware of PR tactics and false experts? Or are those tactics and experts becoming more savvy and effective?

Stauber: The truth is that the situation is getting worse, not better. More and more of what we see, hear and read as "news" is actually PR content. On any given day much or most of what the media transmits or prints as news is provided by the PR industry. It's off press releases, the result of media campaigns, heavily spun and managed, or in the case of "video news releases" it's fake TV news—stories completely produced and supplied for free by former journalists who've gone over to PR. TV news directors air these VNRs as news. So the media not only fails to identify PR manipulations, it is the guilty party by passing them on as news.

Hausman: What's the solution for the excesses of the PR industry? Just more media literacy and watchdog organizations like yours? Or should the PR industry be regulated in some way?

Stauber: In our last chapter, "Question Authority," we identify some of the most common propaganda tactics so that individuals and journalists and public inter-est scientists can do a better job of not being snowed and fooled. But ultimately those who have the most power and money in any society are going to use the most sophisticated propaganda tactics available to keep democracy at bay and the rabble in line.

There are some specific legislative steps that could be taken without stepping on the First Amendment. One is that all nonprofit, tax-exempt organizations—charities and educational groups, for instance—should be required by law to reveal their institutional funders of, say, $500 or more. That way when a journalist or a citizen hears that a scientific report is from a group like the American Council on Science and Health, a quick trip to an IRS Web site could reveal that this group gets massive infusions of industry money, and that the corporations that fund it benefit from its proclamations that pesticides are safe, genetically engineered food will save the planet, lead contamination isn't really such a big deal, climate change isn't happening, and so on. *The public clearly doesn't understand that most nonprofit groups (not ours, by the way) take industry and government grants. Many are even the nonprofit arm of industry.*

Hausman: What led you, personally, to become one of the PR industry's most vocal critics?

Stauber: In 1990 I found myself spied upon by the world's largest PR firm, Burson-Marsteller. I had organized a conference in Washington, D.C., of a couple dozen leaders of farm, consumer, animal welfare and environmental groups all opposed to the FDA's eventual approval of Monsanto's genetically engineered bovine growth hormone, called rBGH.

Now, I personally knew everyone participating, except a young woman who claimed to be with the Maryland Consumers Council, a group of "housewives" who said they wanted to make sure their kids didn't have to drink milk from cows injected with the hormonal drug rBGH. Well, a few months later a reporter called and asked if I knew that Monsanto had a spy in our meeting. I investigated and discovered that the consumer group was phony, that the woman worked for Burson-Marsteller, and that one of B-M's clients was Eli Lilly, who along with Monsanto was one of the developers of rBGH.

I found out that this was typical of corporate PR, and I was outraged at having been spied upon and infiltrated. So I focused my activism onto the PR industry, founded PR Watch in 1993, and it has been very sweet revenge indeed.

If the PR industry doesn't like what we do, they only have themselves to blame for our existence.

Reprinted with permission from Alternet.org

Detroit Metro Times February 6, 2001

Modern Medicine Gets a Failing Grade: Birth of the Lifestyle Approach

Gary Null, PhD

There is no longer a debate about the fact that we are an unhealthy nation. Neither is there a debate about the causes: smoking, unhealthy diet, and lack of physical exercise to name the most obvious. The debate is enjoined when we search for solutions. We expect solutions to come from within our health care system, from the Surgeon General, the CDC, the Department of Health and Welfare. However, it comes as no surprise that there has never been a national health program and no one is giving us important lifestyle direction.

We do have a solution. It's called CLIP, the Comprehensive Lifestyle Intervention Program, a program that has improved the health of people from all over the country, of all ages, and all walks of life. It's a program that involves diet, supplements, exercise, stress reduction, and behavioral counseling. But first let's define the problem.

Death by Cigarettes and Chocolate

The Journal of the American Medical Association (JAMA) is arguably the most prestigious peer reviewed medical journal in the U.S, even in the world. What JAMA says between its covers is state-of-the art medical science. Therefore, in March 2004, when JAMA published the paper *Actual Causes of Death in the United States, 2000*, it was sending a message to the American people.[1]

One of the authors of this paper is none other than Dr. Julie Gerberding, the head of the Centers for Disease Control (CDC), whose name became a household word when she calmed the fears of the American people about the SARS epidemic in 2003. During her long career, Dr. Gerberding has written over 101 medical journal articles since 1985. Another author, Dr. Donna Stroup, has accumulated at least sixty-three journal publications since 1987 and mainly writes extensive medical literature reviews on a wide variety of topics. Dr. J. S. Marks has over 133 journal articles stretching back to 1960 with a focus on public health and lifestyle factors. Dr. Ali Mokdad's fifty-eight papers written since 1994 also follow lifestyle health risks such as obesity, arthritis, diabetes heart disease, and the distribution of measures such as C-reactive protein (a sign of inflammation) in the population.

These four doctors who wrote *Actual Causes of Death in the United States, 2000* are obviously very accomplished researchers and writers, and considering that Dr. Gerberding is head of the CDC, they wield considerable power. The important message they are sending to the American public concerns lifestyle. Echoing what the World Health Organization has been saying for decades, that tobacco and lifestyle are the major causes of death in North America, Gerberding, et al. have quantified these deaths.

We have long been told that heart disease and cancer are the leading causes of death. We are shown these numbers every few years as the epidemic of these chronic diseases escalates. However, Gerberding and her colleagues have not just counted the end result of a lifetime of illness and called it heart disease or cancer. They have quantified the actual causes of disease and labeled them accordingly.

Actual Causes of Death

1. Tobacco	435,000
2. Poor diet and Poor physical inactivity	400,000
3. Alcohol consumption	85,000
4. Infectious agents (e.g., influenza and pneumonia)	75,000
5. Toxic agents (e.g., pollutants and asbestos)	55,000
6. Motor vehicle accidents	43,000
7. Firearms	29,000
8. Sexual behavior	20,000
9. Illicit use of drugs	17,000

The fact that tobacco causes deaths due to cancer, respiratory disease, and chronic infection is nothing new but what is alarming is that, according to this chart in Gerberding's paper, most deaths in the American population are due to tobacco smoking. Even more shocking is the 400,000 deaths due to poor diet and lack of physical activity. The number is a shock and so is the admission. As the so-called richest country in the world, we are admitting that this extraordinary number of people are so malnourished and in such bad physical conditioning that it's killing them.

The World View

Dr. Pekka Puska, Director of the Department of Non-Communicable Disease (NCD) Prevention for the World Health Organization (WHO) presented at a WHO Global Forum on NCD Prevention and Control in Rio de Janeiro, November 9-12, 2003. In his presentation *Working Together for a Healthy Future: Setting the Scene,* he outlined the worldwide causes of death in 2000. The assembly was shocked when he stated that seven out of ten main mortality risk factors are impacted by lifestyle choices. These risk factors, that affect both adults and children include:

1. Blood pressure
2. Tobacco
3. Cholesterol
4. Fruit and vegetable intake
5. Alcohol
6. High BMI
7. Physical Activity

Dr. Puska warned of the emerging epidemic of NCDs that is "to a great extent a consequence of rapid changes in the diets, of declining physical activity and of increase of tobacco use." He emphasized that medical evidence for prevention exists and that population-based prevention is the most cost-effective and the only affordable option for major public health improvement in NCD rates. He said that WHO is making NCD's a priority with an emphasis on prevention. In the case of tobacco, Dr. Puska suggested higher taxes and a comprehensive advertisement ban. Three health programs were also launched.

1. Tobacco: Quit and Win
2. Physical Activity: Move for Health
3. Diet: Global Fruit and Vegetable Initiative

Blame the Victim

It's very important that the CDC and the WHO are admitting that poor diet and lack of exercise is a major concern. Is their concern coming a little too late to help the already millions of sufferers of chronic disease? It shouldn't be forgotten *that alternative medicine and integrative medicine doctors have been harping about this situation for decades.*

Should we, in fact, be suspicious of the timing? After all, President Bush has made the statement that the health care system in America is on a collision course with bankruptcy and has set the date of the final fire sale on our health care for 2011. Perhaps a cynical mind can see the statistics on tobacco and lifestyle as a "blame the victim" ploy. After all, we are the ones that take a drag on the cigarette and Super-Size ourselves on a regular basis.

Morgan Spurlock, the writer, directory, producer, actor, and now nutrition media star, in his own reality drama of a one-month "mac-attack" proved that we are the cause of our own. After one month of a MacDonald's diet he gained twenty-five pounds, had elevated blood levels of cholesterol, triglycerides, liver enzymes, uric acid. He also developed mood swings, depression, fatigue, and apathy.

Preventive Medicine

But let's be positive, perhaps the CDC is finally gearing up their preventive medicine forces because the standard practice of medicine is not working. Evidence of adverse drug reactions, medical mistakes, malnutrition in hospitals and nursing homes, thousands dying of bedsores are all reaching the inevitable crescendo of loss of faith in the "standard practice of care" because the standard practice of care seems to wholly embrace drugs and eschews alternatives in every form.

Dangerous Supplements

Witness the current attempt by the FDA to "control dangerous" supplements. In 2003, Sen. Richard Durbin of Illinois introduced the Supplement Safety Act (S.722) that would treat nutritional supplements like drugs. Let's compare the deaths caused by supplements and those caused by drugs. In a paper published in JAMA in 1998, the authors reported that in American hospitals, in one year alone, **2.2 million people suffered serious adverse effects from properly prescribed drugs, 106,000 died.**[2] Countless others died later, from their injuries. In any given year in America from 0-2 people might die from taking a hefty overdose of a potent herb, rarely, if ever, from taking the prescribed or recommended amount.

Majority of Americans Use Complementary Alternative Medicine (CAM)

CAM is defined as everything that standard medicine is not. So, everything that is not a drug, or surgery, or chemotherapy, or radiation-is CAM. Modern medicine has a monopoly on health care and it is in charge of creating the standards of practice of medicine. CAM is everything else and is routinely reminded that it is the black sheep in the health care family. However, that is not the opinion of the American people in a recent survey.

In a chilling indictment of the "standard practice of medical care," 28 percent of the American adult population is turning to alternative medical and health modalities because they say they no longer have trust or faith in modern medicine.[1] That percentage translates into 79 million disenfranchised citizens that are sufficiently fed up with the "standard practice of medicine" that they are looking for and paying for alternatives. In the words of the authors of a 2004 nationwide study conducted by the CDC and the National Center for Complementary and Alternative Medicine (NCCAM), 28 percent of 31,000 people surveyed admitted that they used CAM because *they believed conventional medical treatments would not help them with their health problem.* The authors found this view was in contrast to previous surveys that CAM users were not, in general, dissatisfied with conventional medicine.

The survey offered the most thorough look at CAM modalities and interviewed a much larger population than ever before. Interviewers met directly with participants and asked questions about twenty-seven types of CAM therapies commonly used in the U.S. Ten therapies were administered by a practitioner such as chiropractic, acupuncture, and massage and the rest involved self-care-diets, herbs, vitamins, minerals, aromatherapy, etc. Thirty-six percent of the individuals surveyed used some form of CAM. This translates into 102 million Americans. When prayer, used specifically for health, was included as a CAM therapy the number rose to 62 percent.

The highest percentage of users of CAM have a higher education; are women; people who had been hospitalized within the past year; and former smokers. The director of the CDC's National Center for Health Statistics (NCHS) Edward J. Sondik, Ph.D. admitted that, "Over the years we've concentrated on traditional medical treatment, (in our surveys) but this new collection of CAM data taps into another dimension entirely. What we see is that a sizable percentage of the public puts their personal health into their own hands."

What a surprise! The researchers were also surprised that "only about 12 percent of adults sought care from a licensed CAM practitioner, suggesting that most people who use CAM do so without consulting a practitioner."

We would suggest that all along a certain segment of the population has been quietly taking care of their own health. Women over the ages have been herbalists, midwives, and caregivers. Then several centuries ago herbalists were targeted as witches, then midwives were no longer allowed to practice without a doctor's supervision and everyone who wanted to help another had to be regulated, read, and controlled by a license. And, it's only in the past 100 years or so that modern medicine has imbued people with the idea that only doctors can diagnose and treat disease and offer a drug or surgery as their only?cure?. We would suggest that many people are waking up to the problems of the standard practice of medicine and taking matters into their own hands.

Drug Companies Lose their Grip

It takes very little imagination to see what is happening with the attack on natural supplements and the recent CAM survey. Pharmaceutical companies make tens of billions of dollars selling drugs and they don't want 36-62 percent of American population relying on CAM instead of a steady diet of drugs.

Is the CDC's Prevention Program Enough to Break the Drug Monopoly?

On the CDC website are CDC's Prevention Activities that Target Actual Causes of Death.?[4]

1. Tobacco: The CDC supports and funds programs all over the country to prevent and control tobacco use. Their most active programs are *Quitline*—telephone-based tobacco cessation services, which include educational materials, referral to local programs, and individualized telephone counseling.

2. Obesity: The CDC supports state nutrition and physical activity programs and currently funds twenty states to *prevent and reduce the prevalence of obesity and the chronic diseases associated with obesity.*

3. Infectious Diseases: The main thrust surveillance and an education program about the overuse of antibiotics called the *Get Smart: Know When Antibiotics Work* campaign.

4. Toxic Agents: The CDC is working to determine which environmental chemicals get into people's bodies and at what levels. It is assessing the effectiveness of public health efforts to reduce people's exposure to specific chemicals. CDC is also tracking trends in levels of people's exposure to environmental chemicals and setting priorities for research on human health effects of exposure to environmental chemicals. CDC is funding schools of public health to support state and local health departments and to investigate possible links between the health and the environment.

Deconstructing the CDC's Prevention Program

What's wrong with the CDC's Prevention Program? It just doesn't go far enough.

Tobacco: Let's look at this sensibly. The CDC on it's own website claims that it "serves as the national focus for developing and applying disease prevention and control, environmental health, and health promotion and education activities designed to improve the health of the people of the United States." The May 2004, Surgeon General's Report on Smoking and Health, expanded the list of diseases caused by tobacco. Dr. Richard H. Carmona revealed for the first time that smoking causes diseases in "nearly every organ of the body." We've known for many years that smoking causes cancer, heart disease, and strokes but this newest report finds that cigarette smoking "is conclusively linked to diseases such as leukemia, cataracts, pneumonia, and cancers of the cervix, kidney, pancreas and stomach."

As with DDT, and as with almost every toxic chemical that has been tested over the past several decades we have some official saying exactly what Dr. Carmona says about smoking "We've known for decades that smoking is bad for your health, but this report shows that it's even worse than we knew. The toxins from cigarette smoke go everywhere the blood flows."

According to a Department of Health and Human Services report on smoking, on average, men who smoke cut their lives short by 13.2 years, and female smokers lose 14.5 years. The economic toll exceeds $157 billion each year in the

United States—$75 billion in direct medical costs and $82 billion in lost productivity. Knowing all this, if you were in charge of the CDC, wouldn't you want to do a little more to curb tobacco smoking in our population?

Obesity: Unfortunately schools are supported by soft drink companies that sell soda in schools adding to the rate of obesity in children. By allowing sugar to comprise up to 25 percent of the dietary calories, for children, adolescents, and young people, we will continue to have the highest rate of obesity in the world.

Infectious Diseases: Nowhere in the recommendations about preventing infectious disease is there mention of alternatives to antibiotics. Even though there are natural antibiotics such as garlic and colloidal silver, which have been scientifically proven to kill many pathogens, the CDC continues to promote the notion that there is no other treatment for infections but antibiotics.

Toxic Agents: To say that the CDC has a prevention program for toxic agents is disingenuous. They merely continue to collect data. They make no mention of the 100,000 chemicals in existence or the fact that few of them have passed safety tests, and the fact that most of those, when they are tested are found to be carcinogenic.

Sugar and Health

In the report *Actual Causes of Death* 34 percent of U.S. adults are considered overweight, and an additional 31 percent are obese. In 2001, chronic diseases contributed approximately 59% of the 56.5 million total reported deaths in the world and 46% of the global burden of disease. Yet, the sugar industry will not admit that sugar has anything to do with causing weight, heart disease, or cancer. The most it will admit to is that sugar can cause cavities, but then all you need to do is take a poisonous chemical called fluoride and rub that on your teeth "but not swallow it" and you will be just fine.

The sugar industry is currently lobbying congress to stop funding the UN because of a UN health recommendation to reduce the amount of calories in the world's diet. Presently, U.S. diet recommendations allow 25 percent of calories to come from sugar! Imagine four meals in one day, three square and one snack, but mix them all up and take 1/4 of that amount and make it all sugar. That is what most young people are eating-up to 40 teaspoons of sugar a day. Estimates of sugar consumption say that every American consumes an annual 150 pounds of sugar. These are the facts we need to learn. However, as long as the sugar industry controls the government and won't allow the proper nutrition education, we will continue to be a Super-Sized nation.

Thirty international experts, commissioned by two U.N. agencies, the World Health Organization (WHO) and the Food and Agriculture Organization (FAO) came out with a new report. It's called The Joint WHO/FAO Expert Report, Diet, Nutrition and the Prevention of Chronic Disease. The experts agree that it's time that people limited their sugar intake to no more than 10 percent of calories. They also crossed that imaginary line in the sand when they said that cutting back on sugar would help put the brakes on the global epidemic of obesity-related disease. The UN is coming out against sugar and therefore against the sugar industry.

USA Today reported that the sugar industry is criticizing the document, refuting once again that sugar affects weight. The US National Soft Drink Association made the oft heard claim that the "scientific literature does not show an association between sugar intake and obesity." They just don't recognize the fact that all Americans are *the experiment* and the results are obvious. The sugar industry is making their own health recommendation that exercise is what Americans are lacking. Actually, the UN report did advise twice as much exercise as the US guidelines, one hour instead of thirty minutes as well as a deep cut in sugar.[5]

The CDC and Chronic Disease

Nowhere in the CDC Prevention Activities does it mention the need to curb chronic disease. However, the CDC has it's own Chronic Disease Prevention website and chronic disease programs that "provide national leadership by offering guidelines and recommendations and by helping state health and education agencies promote healthy behaviors."[6] The CDC is all in favor of promoting health behaviors but there are no recommendations for detoxification programs, an organic diet, or nutritional supplements. Looking at their specific programs it's all about measuring data, screening for disease, and using billions of dollars in the process. The CDC overview of chronic disease makes their lack of aggressive treatment and prevention chilling.[7] The CDC says that "Today, chronic diseases such as cardiovascular disease (primarily heart disease and stroke), cancer, and diabetes are among the most prevalent, costly, and preventable of all health problems. Seven of every 10 Americans who die each year, which is more than 1.7 million people, succumb to chronic disease."

The Cost of Chronic Disease

The CDC admits that the "United States cannot effectively address escalating health care costs without addressing the problem of chronic diseases." The following stunning statistics are taken from the CDC?s Chronic Disease Overview:[8]

1. More than 90 million Americans live with chronic illnesses.

2. Chronic diseases account for 70% of all deaths in the United States.

3. The medical care costs of people with chronic diseases account for more than 75% of the nation's $1.4 trillion annual medical care costs.

4. Chronic diseases account for one-third of the years of potential life lost before age 65.

5. Hospitalizations for pregnancy-related complications occurring before delivery account for more than $1 billion annually.

6. The direct and indirect costs of diabetes are nearly $132 billion a year.

7. Each year, arthritis results in estimated medical care costs of more than $22 billion, and estimated total costs (medical care and lost productivity) of almost $82 billion.

8. The estimated direct and indirect costs associated with smoking exceed $75 billion annually.

9. In 2001, approximately $300 billion was spent on all cardiovascular diseases. Over $129 billion in lost productivity was due to cardiovascular disease.

10. The direct medical costs associated with physical inactivity was nearly $76.6 billion in 2000.

11. Nearly $68 billion is spent on dental services each year.

The Lifestyle Approach

WHO and FAO hope their Report on Diet and Chronic Disease findings will provide member states with enough ammunition to prepare national health strategies. Dr. Richard Uauy, lead author of the report made a number of astute observations.[9]

Dr. Uauy said that

1. "Not all fats or all carbohydrates are the same; it pays to know the difference."

2. "People should eat less high-calorie foods, especially foods high in saturated fat and sugar, be physically active, prefer unsaturated for saturated fat and use less salt; enjoy fruits, vegetables and legumes and prefer foods of plant and marine origin."

3. "A diet rich in fruit and vegetables containing immune-system boosting micronutrients could also help the body's natural defenses against infectious diseases."

The specific recommendations on diet are as follows:

1. Limit fat to between 15 and 30 percent of total daily energy

2. Limit saturated fats to less than 10 percent of this total fat consumer

3. Carbohydrates provide the bulk of energy requirements between 55 and 75 percent of daily intake.

4. Free sugars should remain beneath 10 percent.

5. Protein should make up a further 10-15 percent of calorie intake.

6. Salt should be restricted to less than 5 grams a day.

7. Intake of fruit and vegetables should reach at least 400 grams a day (about 14 ounces).

The report warns that obesity is not the only factor of concern with a poor diet but that chronic disease, such as hypertension and heart disease are caused by a diet high in saturated fats and excess salt. The amount of exercise recommended by the UN report is double the amount suggested in the US. One full hour a day of *moderate-intensity activity, such as walking,* as many days as possible is said to be needed to maintain a healthy body weight. Unlike the CDC preventive activities, the WHO/FAO report does recognize chronic disease as a prevalent but preventable problem, which is directly related to diet and exercise. The importance of creating an environment that supports health is also stressed.

Comprehensive Lifestyle Intervention Program (CLIP)

One of the only programs that comes close to the recommendations of the WHO/FAO has been tested over the past twelve years in the U.S. on thousands of participants. CLIP, conducted over a six month or a twelve month period, is an analysis of whether comprehensive lifestyle changes lead to improvement in several parameters: heart disease risk factors, obesity, symptoms of arthritis, menopause symptoms, and general health.

CLIP consists of a diverse group of individuals, including those who wish to maintain their health and those who are suffering from one or more illnesses. A total of 11,214 people participated in CLIP over a span of twelve years. The protocols involved comprehensive lifestyle changes non-calorie-restricted whole foods vegetarian and fish diet, supplements, aerobic exercise, resistance exercise, stress management, and two-hour weekly meetings, which included behavior modification. These protocols were implemented and participants were followed, sometimes for several years, after completion of their protocol.

The following objective data was collected from participants, first when the entered the program and when they graduated: cholesterol, LDL cholesterol, cholesterol/HDL ratio, homocysteine, blood pressure, weight, and impedance. Subjective data from participants consisted of daily journals and formatted questionnaires covering weight loss, menopause, arthritis, fatigue, aging, hair loss, anxiety/depression, and men's health.

Analysis of data from the study was able to determine that adherence to intensive lifestyle changes showed improvement in blood tests, physical exams, and health scores. The participants' detailed questionnaires showed improvements in nine different physical and mental functions and specific disease symptoms rated on a scale of 1 to 10. Markers included: energy, endurance, immune system function (catching colds etc.), mental function (memory, concentration), sugar problems (craving carbohydrates, hypoglycemia), skin (changes), joints, digestion, and hair.

Laboratory and clinical data revealed the following average reductions: a reduction of 16.3 percent in blood homocysteine levels; a reduction of 10.7 percent in total cholesterol; a reduction of 5.3 percent in LDL; a reduction of 10.3 percent in total cholesterol/HDL; an 11.6 percent reduction in systolic blood pressure, and a 13.8 percent reduction in diastolic blood pressure.

Researchers implementing CLIP were able to demonstrate that a comprehensive lifestyle intervention approach offers a safe and healthy way to lower cholesterol, homocysteine, blood pressure, and weight, and enhance overall general wellness, with no adverse side effects.

Because the focus of CLIP is on a comprehensive approach, including many different interventions, we did not measure the effect of each individual nutrient or lifestyle change. It is difficult, if not impossible, to measure scientifically, the power of individual causes in a lifestyle study. In implementing CLIP we chose to do what very few studies have done before. We chose to incorporate a totality of lifestyle changes that we felt could impact the progression of disease and enhancement of wellness and measure their overall effect.

In background research we recognized that large survey studies like the 122,000-person Nurses Health Study don't give definitive answers about health and neither are they double-blind, cross over.[10] For example, the Nurses Health Study published the following conclusion—by consuming an extra two pieces of fruit per week you can lower your risk of acquiring a particular disease by a certain percentage. But, how do we know that consuming the two extra pieces of fruit per week were a cause, and not a coincidental factor, among many factors, that led to lower risk of acquiring the particular disease? The answer is that with such large survey studies, we do not know with scientific precision what constitutes a cause of a particular health condition and what may just be a coincidental effect. Yet, this lack of precision as to the determination of cause and effect does not render these studies meaningless. Instead, they are helpful to the extent that they demonstrate important correlations that may be further studied.

Lifestyle

Americans are increasingly overweight, fatigued, and suffer multiple types of pain, which diminishes their quality of life. The concept of lifestyle intervention is becoming more common in the literature.[11-20] This study did not address any specific illnesses, rather its focus was on the outcome of major changes in a person's lifestyle and environment. Therefore, diet, supplements, exercise, stress management, behavior modification, and making an environmentally safer work and home environment were the main variables.

The following background information on cholesterol, blood pressure, obesity, and chronic disease serves to emphasize why CLIP is not directed at any particular disease, but at an epidemic of disease and bad health.

Cholesterol Facts

One-third of Americans have borderline-high risk cholesterol levels. Coronary heart disease (CHD) is the leading cause of death in America and high cholesterol levels contribute to the incidence of this disease. According to the American Heart Association borderline-high risk cholesterol levels are between 200-239 mg/dl.21 Desirable cholesterol is below 200 mg/dl and optimum LDL is below 100 mg/dl.22, 23 and the optimum ratio of cholesterol to HDL is 3.5:1.[24]

Blood Pressure Facts

According to the American Heart Association, one in four Americans have high blood pressure and one-third of those are unaware that they do.25 The Seventh Report of the Joint National Committee on Prevention, Detection, Evaluation, and Treatment of High Blood Pressure presented its guidelines for doctors in a JAMA article.26 The following are some highlights from the JAMA article.

1. The risk of cardiovascular disease, beginning at 115/75 mm Hg, doubles with each increment of 20/10 mm Hg.

2. People who have normal blood pressure at 55 years of age have a 90% lifetime risk for developing hypertension.

3. People with a systolic BP of 120 to 139 mm Hg or a diastolic BP of 80 to 89 mm Hg should be considered as pre-hypertensive and require health-promoting lifestyle modifications to prevent CVD.

Homocysteine Facts

In 1998 the American Medical Association's (AMA) Council of Scientific Affairs addressed the relationship of folic acid, vitamins B6, B12, and homocysteine; folic acid and vitamin B12 deficiency and potential risk factors for cardiovascular and Alzheimer's disease; and folate and colorectal cancer in Report 8. Also in 1998, feeling an urgency to investigate homocysteine, the AMA "encouraged the CDC and the NIH to fund basic and epidemiological studies and clinical trials to determine causal and metabolic relationships among homocysteine, vitamins B12 and B6, and folic acid, so as to reduce the risks for and incidence of associated diseases and deficiency states." The AMA also urged the FDA to increase folic acid fortification to 350?g per 100 g of enriched cereal grain.[27] There has been no update on homocysteine since 1998 but it continues to be a topic of considerable research activity.[28-36]

Chronic Disease Facts

Several major chronic diseases are greatly impacted by environmental and lifestyle factors. According to the American Heart Association, approximately 61.8 million people suffer from cardiovascular disease, which includes hypertension, heart diseases, and stroke.[37] A 2003 study released by the Centers for Disease Control and Prevention (CDC) revealed that since 1997, the incidence of arthritis has soared from 43 million to 70 million. Therefore, at least one out of every three adults in the United States suffers from arthritis and/or chronic joint symptoms. The CEO of the Arthritis Foundation said that, "We are a nation in pain. Arthritis is the number one cause of disability and affects more people than ever imagined."[38]

Obesity Facts

According to the Centers for Disease Control (CDC), "Obesity has risen at an epidemic rate during the past 20 years."[39] The CDC says that in 2003, the number of obese Americans is 44 million. In 2000, 64% of U.S. adults were overweight or obese. Fifteen percent of adolescents and children were also overweight. A Rand Corporation study published in October, 2003, shows that for the years 1986-2000, an alarming 1 in 50 Americans are 100 pounds overweight or more. The number of morbidly obese Americans has thus risen dramatically from its 1986 level of only 1 in 200. What was thought to be a rare group of overweight individuals, who are 150 pounds or more overweight, is becoming more common. That group grew from 1 in 2,000 Americans to 1 in 400 during the same 14-year study period.[40]

Metabolic Syndrome Facts

The health impact of obesity becomes obvious when addressing the condition called "metabolic syndrome." A 2002 JAMA study estimates that 47 million Americans may exhibit this syndrome characterized by insulin resistance, obesity, abdominal fat, high blood sugar, high triglycerides, high blood cholesterol, and high blood pressure.[41] Editorializing on this study the CDC advises that, "Because the root causes of the metabolic syndrome for a majority of individuals may be poor diet and insufficient physical activity, the high prevalence of the syndrome underscores an urgent need to develop comprehensive efforts directed at controlling the U.S. obesity epidemic and improving physical activity levels within the U.S. population."[42]

The intent of CLIP is to provide a diet, exercise, supplements, and lifestyle intervention program for preventing and reversing heart disease, arthritis, obesity, and the metabolic syndrome.

One Example of the Importance of Nutrients

Time and space does not permit an in depth description of specific nutrients but we offer one example of the importance of a group of nutrients in disease improvement and wellness. Other areas of nutrient research, such as antioxidant nutrition, essential fatty acids, or amino acids have similar bodies of evidence and will be a topic for a future paper.

Researchers have found that simple, food-based, methyl groups that are components of common nutrients—folic acid, choline, B-12, and B-6—can turn on or off genes. During methylation, a methyl group attaches to a gene at a specific point and induces changes in the way the gene is expressed.[43] In one very important study with implications for pregnant women and their offspring, a diet rich in methyl groups (folic acid, choline, B-12, and B-6) turned off a gene that led to adult obesity and diabetes in mice. Methyl groups are entirely derived from the foods people eat; they include vitamin B12, folic acid, choline, and betaine from sugar beets.[44]

Interestingly, these same nutrients, folic acid, B-12 and B-6 have a role to play in preventing heart disease. A genetic weakness in the body's ability to lower the levels of the amino acid homocysteine has been linked to premature vascular disease. These nutrients prevent homocysteine build up and consequent heart disease by changing homocysteine to the safer amino acid, methionine.

Risk Factor Analysis

The state of the art in assessing risk factors contributing to disease began with the Framingham Heart Study (1948), followed by the all-female, Nurses Health Study (1976), and the all-male Health Professionals Follow-Up Study (1986). Hundreds of journal articles have flourished from excavating reams of statistics compiled every two years in these surveys consisting of tens of thousands of people. Over time, as the number of participants succumb to a particular disease, those who were inflicted with the disease are compared in numerous ways with those who were not. The limitations of such studies are considerable. Manipulating the statistics of such large numbers of people (the original Nurses Health Study enrolled 122,000) makes the final results appear impressive. However, nutritional data compiled from diet histories alone may be insufficient to tell us enough about a specific nutrient to determine true risk reduction.

Human and animal short-term nutrient studies done on one nutrient at a time merely show that a specific nutrient deficiency contributes to symptoms and a specific nutrient replacement may modify those symptoms. But, isolating one symptom and treating it with one nutrient in a simple cause and effect approach should not be our only criteria for understanding the role of nutrients in health. We believe that by examining the human in the larger context of their life, including diet, supplement intake, exercise status, and stress reduction, is much more relevant and can be examined statistically using the objective and subjective measures that we have chosen.

Specific Dietary Requirements:

- A mostly, non-caloric-restricted (people were not limited to a certain number of calories) vegetarian diet which included fish, soybeans and soy products, quinoa (high protein grain), mixed grains and beans, soy isoflavone or rice protein powder drinks (20 grams three times a day).

- From six to nine servings of fruits and vegetables a day, Four servings of beans and whole grains such as whole brown rice, millet, oats, barley, kamut, amaranth, quinoa, spelt.

- Two servings of starchy vegetables per day, such as kohlrabi, turnips, squash.

- One whole onion and a 1/2 bulb of garlic a day.

- One serving of sea vegetables a day.

- Four ounces of fresh organic vegetable juice diluted with 4 oz of water building up gradually to six times a day. Most vegetables were used including celery, cucumber, beet, cabbage and could include apple for taste, and several ounces of aloe vera juice per day.

Specific Nutrient Supplementation

The total daily intake of nutrients was as follows. The selection of nutrients was based on a literature review of over 50,000 journal articles showing positive health indications for these supplements.

- Vitamin B1—25 mg
- Vitamin B2—25 mg

- Vitamin B6—50 mg

- Vitamin B12—1,000 micrograms

- Folic Acid—800 micrograms

- Biotin—100 micrograms

- Pantothenic acid—100 mg

- PABA—100 mg

- Niacin—100 mg

- Calcium and magnesium—1,000mg

- Chromium—200 micrograms

- Selenium—200 micrograms

- Vitamin D—400 IU

- Vitamin E—400 IU

- Vitamin C—5,000 mg

- Choline and inositol—100 mg

- L-Carnosine—500 mg

- Coenzyme Q10—200 mg

- TMG—400 mg

Exercise

Participants gradually increased their level of activity to one hour a day with 1/2 hour resistance training (weight training) and 1/2 hour general aerobic training. Power walking was offered as one of the best ways to get aerobic exercise. Power walking is basically walking very fast, always with one foot on the ground, to maintain cardiovascular health and burn calories.

Behavior Modification

We took the "no more excuses" approach in the form of detailed journaling of day-to-day life issues and challenges. At each weekly session people were able to discuss their problems and shared solutions with each other with input from professionals. In group discussions participants learned to identify their sublimation of choice, whether it was overworking, complaining, overeating, drug taking, gambling, or sex, and sought to modify this behavior. Specific behavior modification educators in the mass media such as Norman Cousins, Wayne Dwyer, George Leonard and Herbert Benson were models for this part of CLIP and their books were recommended reading. [145-148]

Stress Management

Stress management consisted of two 1/2 hour sessions per day of prayer, meditation, journal writing, listening to calming music, walking, yoga, tai chi, or any other soothing, de-stressing technique.

Environment

Participants were instructed to clean up their living and work environments, remove toxins such as paint thinners, pesticides, and strong cleaning products, and obtain air and water filtration systems.

Results of a Lifestyle Approach

The total number of participants enrolled in CLIP over a ten-year period was 11,124. The percentage of participants who were not able to complete the program was 36 percent.

Blood Pressure

We found that not only could we modify blood pressure in the pre-hypertensive range, but also in the hypertensive range, and without resorting to anti-hypertensive medications. The average drop in systolic pressure was 12 percent and the average drop in diastolic pressure was 14 percent.

Cholesterol

The average reduction of total cholesterol for all three groups was 10.7 percent. The average reduction in LDL cholesterol was 15.3 percent.

Homocysteine

Homocysteine is a relatively new, but very important marker for heart disease that we have only been measuring since 2001, and only in our Open Groups. The following represents preliminary data collection on all participants. There was an average of 16.3% reduction in homocysteine levels with consistently greater reduction for subjects who began the study with levels 11.5 units or greater.

Targeted Groups

From 1990-1999 all participants were only entered into Open Groups. From 1999-2003 there were Open Groups and Targeted Groups. Targeted Groups consisted of participants with specific disease criteria confirmed by a doctor's letter. In these groups, there was an average 82 percent improvement in health parameters for people who completed their program. People lost weight-in some cases over 150 pounds; arthritis sufferers eliminated their pain and were taken off their medication; those with fatigue got their energy back; women with menopause no longer had symptoms; seniors slowed down the aging process; men improved their libido and reversed impotence; people with mood disorders greatly decreased their symptoms of anxiety and depression and were often taken off their medications. At the routine six-months follow up 73 percent continued to have sustained improvement and did not relapse into past bad habits and behaviors. They acknowledged how easy it was to maintain their lifestyle. People continued to report that they felt extremely well. Those who lost up to 100 pounds maintained their weight loss.

The CLIP results clearly show that a conscientious shift toward healthier lifestyle choices: diet, supplements, exercise, behavior modification, and stress reduction can make a difference in health outcome. CLIP provides proof that lifestyle modification is able to change biochemistry and physical and mental symptoms, and disease symptoms in many individuals. CLIP also shows that health improvement is possible in a diverse group of individuals who are making incremental adjustments to their daily routine. Not only was change possible in people who presented with disease conditions but CLIP provided relatively healthy people with the tools to maintain wellness.

Reprinted with Permission from Gary Null and Associates

REFERENCES

1. Mokdad AH, Marks JS, Stroup DF, Gerberding JL. Actual causes of death in the United States, 2000. JAMA. 2004 Mar 10;291(10):1238-45.)

2. Lazarou J, Pomeranz B, Corey P. Incidence of adverse drug reactions in hospitalized patients. JAMA. 1998;279:1200-1205.

3. http://nccam.nih.gov/news/camsurvey.htm

4. http://www.cdc.gov/nccdphp/factsheets/death_causes2000.htm

5. USA Today, March 2, 2004. London AP. http://www.usatoday.com/news/health/2003-03-02-world-sugar_x.htm

6. http://www.cdc.gov/nccdphp/overview.htm

7. Ibib

8. http://www.cdc.gov/nccdphp/overview.htm

9. Food & Agriculture Organization of the United Nations April 23, 2003

10. http://www.channing.harvard.edu/nhs/index.html. Nurses Health Study.

11. Wadden TA, McGuckin BG, Rothman RA, Sargent SL. Lifestyle modification in the management of obesity. J Gastrointest Surg. 2003 May Jun;7(4):452-63.

12. Rock CL, Demark-Wahnefried W. Can lifestyle modification increase survival in women diagnosed with breast cancer? J Nutr. 2002 Nov;132(11 Suppl):3504S-3507S. Review.

13. Song R, Lee H. Effects of a 12-week cardiac rehabilitation exercise program on motivation and health-promoting lifestyle. Heart Lung. 2001 May-Jun;30(3):200-9.

14. Norman RJ, Davies MJ, Lord J, Moran LJ. The role of lifestyle modification in polycystic ovary syndrome. Trends Endocrinol Metab. 2002 Aug;13(6):251-7. Review.

15. Wierenga ME, Oldham KK. Weight control: a lifestyle-modification model for improving health. Nurs Clin North Am. 2002 Jun;37(2):303-13, vii.

16. Davis MM, Jones DW. The role of lifestyle management in the overall treatment plan for prevention and management of hypertension. Semin Nephrol. 2002 Jan;22(1):35-43. Review

17. Wing RR, et al. Behavioral science research in diabetes: lifestyle changes related to obesity, eating behavior, and physical activity. Diabetes Care. 2001 Jan;24(1):117-23. Review.

18. Sevick MA, Dunn AL, Morrow MS, Marcus BH, Chen GJ, Blair SN. Cost-effectiveness of lifestyle and structured exercise interventions in sedentary adults: results of project ACTIVE. Am J Prev Med. 2000 Jul;19(1):1-8.

19. Riebe D, Greene GW, Ruggiero L, Stillwell KM, Blissmer B, Nigg CR, Caldwell M. Evaluation of a healthy-lifestyle approach to weight management. Prev Med. 2003 Jan;36(1):45-54.

20. Frost G, Lyons F, Bovill-Taylor C, Carter L, Stuttard J, Dornhorst A. Intensive lifestyle intervention combined with the choice of pharmacotherapy improves weight loss and cardiac risk factors in the obese. J Hum Nutr Diet. 2002 Aug;15(4):287-95; quiz 297-9.

21. American Heart Association website: http://www.americanheart. org/presenter.jhtml?identifier=1520

22. McKenney JM. Update on the National Cholesterol Education Program Adult Treatment Panel III guidelines: getting to goal. Pharmacotherapy. 2003 Sep;23(9 Pt 2):26S-33S.

23. National Cholesterol Education Program. Third Report of the Expert Panel on Detection, Evaluation, and Treatment of High Blood Cholesterol in Adults (Adult Treatment Panel III) http://www.nhlbi.nih.gov/guidelines/cholesterol/

24. American Heart Association website: http://www.americanheart. org/presenter.jhtml?identifier=4503

25. http://www.americanheart.org/presenter.jhtml?identifier=2114

26. Chobanian AV, et al; National Heart, Lung, and Blood Institute Joint National Committee on Prevention, Detection, Evaluation, and Treatment of High Blood Pressure; National High Blood Pressure Education Program Coordinating Committee. The Seventh Report of the Joint National Committee on Prevention, Detection, Evaluation, and Treatment of High Blood Pressure: the JNC 7 report. JAMA. 2003 May 21;289(19):2560-72.

27. American Medical Association, Report 8 of the Council on Scientific Affairs (A-99) Review of AMA Recommendations on Folic Acid Supplementation. http://www.ama-assn.org/ama/pub/article/2036-2504.html

28. Lee BJ, Lin PT, Liaw YP, Chang SJ, Cheng CH, Huang YC. Homocysteine and risk of coronary artery disease: Folate is the important determinant of plasma homocysteine concentration. Nutrition. 2003 Jul-Aug;19(7-8):577-83.

29. Becker A, Kostense PJ, Bos G, Heine RJ, Dekker JM, Nijpels G, Bouter LM, Stehouwer CD. Hyperhomocysteinaemia is associated with coronary events in type 2 diabetes. J Intern Med. 2003 Mar;253(3):293-300.

30. O'Connor JJ, Meurer LN. Should patients with coronary disease and high homocysteine take folic acid? J Fam Pract. 2003 Jan;52(1):16-8.

31. Remacha AF, Souto JC, Ramila E, Perea G, Sarda MP, Fontcuberta J. Enhanced risk of thrombotic disease in patients with acquired vitamin B12 and/or folate deficiency: role of hyperhomocysteinemia. Ann Hematol. 2002 Nov;81(11):616-21.

32. Woo KS, Qiao M, Chook P, Poon PY, Chan AK, Lau JT, Fung KP, Woo JL. Homocysteine, endothelial dysfunction, and coronary artery disease: emerging strategy for secondary prevention. J Card Surg. 2002 Sep-Oct;17(5):432-5.

33. Romagnuolo J, Fedorak RN, Dias VC, Bamforth F, Teltscher M. Hyperhomocysteinemia and inflammatory bowel disease: prevalence and predictors in a cross-sectional study. Am J Gastroenterol. 2001 Jul;96(7):2143-9.

34. Blum A, Lupovitch S, Khazim K, Peleg A, Gumanovsky M, Yeganeh S, Jawabreh S. Homocysteine levels in patients with risk factors for atherosclerosis. Clin Cardiol. 2001 Jun;24(6):463-6.

35. Blom HJ. Consequences of homocysteine export and oxidation in the vascular system. Seminars in Thrombosis and Haemostasis, 2000;26:227-32.

36. Nyg O et al. Total homocysteine and cardiovascular disease. J Internal Medicine, 1999;246:425-54.

37. http://www.americanheart.org/presenter.jhtml?identifier=3002595

38. Arthritis Foundation Press Release. A New Sense of Urgency About Arthritis: One in Three Adults is Affected. June 11, 2003 http://www.arthritis.org/resources/news/cdc_prevalence_numbers.asp

39. http://www.cdc.gov/nccdphp/dnpa/obesity/index.htm

40. http://www.rand.org/hot/press. 03/10.13.html, Oct. 13, 2003.

41. Ford ES, Giles WH, Dietz WH. Prevalence of the metabolic syndrome among US adults: findings from the third National Health and Nutrition Examination Survey. JAMA. 2002 Jan 16;287(3):356-9.

42. http://www.cdc.gov/nccdphp/dnpa/obesity/trend/metabolic.htm

43. Jones PA, Takai D. The role of DNA methylation in mammalian epigenetics. Science. 2001 Aug 10;293(5532):1068-70.

44. Cooney CA, Dave AA, Wolff GL. Maternal methyl supplements in mice affect epigenetic variation and DNA methylation of offspring. J Nutr. 2002 Aug;132(8 Suppl):2393S-2400S.

The Drug Story

Hans Ruesch

In the 30's, Morris A. Bealle, a former city editor of the old Washington Times and Herald, was running a county seat newspaper, in which the local power company bought a large advertisement every week. This account took quite a lot of worry off Bealle's shoulders when the bills came due.

But according to Bealle's own story, one day the paper took up the cudgels for some of its readers that were being given poor service from the power company, and Morris Bealle received the dressing down of his life from the advertising agency which handled the power company's account. They told him that any more such "stepping out of line" would result in the immediate cancellation not only of the advertising contract, but also of the gas company and the telephone company.

That's when Bealle's eyes were opened to the meaning of a "free press," and he decided to get out of the newspaper business. He could afford to do that because he belonged to the landed gentry of Maryland, but not all newspaper editors are that lucky.

Bealle used his professional experience to do some deep digging into the freedom-of-the-press situation and came up with two shattering exposes—"The Drug Story," and "The House of Rockefeller." The fact that in spite of his familiarity with the editorial world and many important personal contacts he couldn't get his revelations into print until he founded his own company, The Columbia Publishing House, Washington D.C., in 1949, was just a prime example of the silent but adamant censorship in force in "the Land of the Free and the Home of the Brave". Although The Drug Story is one of the most important books on health and politics ever to appear in the USA, it has never been admitted to a major bookstore nor reviewed by any establishment paper, and was sold exclusively by mail. Nevertheless, when we first got to read it, in the 1970s, it was already in its 33rd printing, under a different label—Biworld Publishers, Orem, Utah.

EXAMPLES

As Bealle pointed out, a business which makes 6% on its invested capital is considered a sound money maker. Sterling Drug, Inc., the main cog and largest holding company in the Rockefeller Drug Empire and its 68 subsidiaries, showed operating profits in 1961 of $23,463,719 after taxes, on net assets of $43,108,106—a **54% profit**. Squibb, another Rockefeller-controlled company, in 1945 made not 6% but **576%** on the actual value of its property.

That was during the luscious war years when the Army Surgeon General's Office and the Navy Bureau of Medicine and Surgery were not only acting as promoters for the Drug Trust, but were actually forcing drug trust poisons into the blood streams of American soldiers, sailors and marines, to the tune of over 200 million 'shots.' Is it any wonder, asked Bealle, that the Rockefellers, and their stooges in the Food and Drug Administration, the U.S.

Public Health Service, the Federal Trade Commission, the Better Business Bureau, the Army Medical Corps, the Navy Bureau of Medicine, and thousands of health officers all over the country, should combine to put out of business all forms of therapy that discourage the use of drugs.

"The last annual report of the Rockefeller Foundation," reported Bealle, "itemizes the gifts it has made to colleges and public agencies in the past 44 years, and they total somewhat over half a billion dollars. These colleges, of course, teach their students all the drug lore the Rockefeller pharmaceutical houses want taught. Otherwise there would be no more gifts, just as there are no gifts to any of the 30 odd colleges in the United States that don't use therapies based on drugs."

"Harvard, with its well-publicized medical school, has received $8,764,433 of Rockefeller's Drug Trust money, Yale got $7,927,800, Johns Hopkins $10,418,531, Washington University in St. Louis $2,842,132, New York's Columbia University $5,424,371, Cornell University $1,709,072, etc., etc."

And while "giving away" those huge sums to drug-propagandizing colleges, the Rockefeller interests were growing to a world-wide web that no one could entirely explore. Already well over 30 years ago it was large enough for Bealle to demonstrate that the Rockefeller interests had created, built up and developed the most far reaching industrial empire ever conceived in the mind of man. Standard Oil was of course the foundation upon which all of the other Rockefeller industries have been built. The story of Old John D., as ruthless an industrial pirate as ever came down the pike, is well known, but is being today conveniently ignored. The keystone of this mammoth industrial empire was the *Chase National Bank*, now renamed the *Chase Manhattan Bank*.

Not the least of its holdings are in the drug business. *The Rockefellers own the largest drug manufacturing combine in the world*, and use all of their other interests to bring pressure to increase the sale of drugs. The fact that most of the 12,000 separate drug items on the market are harmful is of no concern to the Drug Trust…

THE ROCKEFELLER FOUNDATION

The Rockefeller Foundation was first set up in 1904 and called the General Education Fund. An organization called the Rockefeller Foundation, ostensibly to supplement the General Education Fund, was formed in 1910 and through long finagling and lots of Rockefeller money got the New York legislature to issue a charter on May 14, 1913.

It is therefore not surprising that the House of Rockefeller has had its own "nominees" planted in all Federal agencies that have to do with health. So the stage was set for the "education" of the American public, with a view to turning it into a population of drug and medico dependents, with the early help of the parents and the schools, then with direct advertising and, last but not least, the influence the advertising revenues had on the media-makers.

A compilation of the magazine *Advertising Age* showed that as far back as 1948 the larger companies in America spent for advertising the sum total of $1,104,224,374, when the dollar was still worth a dollar and not half a zloty. Of this staggering sum the interlocking Rockefeller-Morgan interests (gone over entirely to Rockefeller after Morgan's death) controlled about 80 percent, and utilized it to manipulate public information on health and drug matters—then and even more recklessly now.

CENSORSHIP

"Even the most independent newspapers are dependent on their press associations for their national news," Bealle pointed out, "and there is no reason for a news editor to suspect that a story coming over the wires of the Associated Press, the United Press or the International News Service is censored when it concerns health matters. Yet this is what happens constantly."

In fact in the 50s the Drug Trust had one of its directors on the *directorate of the Associated Press*. He was no less than *Arthur Hays Sulzberger*, publisher of the *New York Times* and as such one of the most powerful Associated Press directors.

It was thus easy for the Rockefeller Trust to persuade the Associated Press Science Editor to adopt a policy which would not permit any medical news to clear that is not approved by the Drug Trust "expert," and this censor is not going to approve any item that can in any way hurt the sale of drugs.

This accounts to this day for the many fake stories of serums and medical cures and just-around-the-corner breakthrough victories over cancer, AIDS, diabetes, multiple sclerosis, which go out brazenly over the wires to all daily newspapers in America and abroad.

Emanuel M. Josephson, M.D., whom the Drug Trust has been unable to intimidate despite many attempts, pointed out that the *National Association of Science Writers* was "persuaded" to adopt as part of its code of ethics the following chestnut: "*Science editors are incapable of judging the facts of phenomena involved in medical and scientific discovery. Therefore, they only report 'discoveries' approved by medical authorities, or those presented before a body of scientific peers.*"

This explains why Bantam Books, America's biggest publisher, made a colossal mistake in its initial enthusiasm and optimism sending review copies of SLAUGHTER OF THE INNOCENT to the 3,500 "science writers" on its list, instead of addressing them to the literary book reviewers who are not subject to medical censorship. One single censor decreed NO and SLAUGHTER OF THE INNOCENT sank in silence.

Thus newspapers continue to be fed with propaganda about drugs and their alleged value, although according to the Food and Drug Administration (FDA) 1.5 million people landed in hospitals in 1978 because of medication side effects in the U.S. alone, and despite recurrent statements by intelligent and courageous medical men that most pharmaceutical items on sale are useless at best, but more often harmful or deadly in the long run.

The truth about cures without drugs is suppressed, unless it suits the purpose of the censor to garble it. Whether these cures are effected by Chiropractors, Naturopaths, Naprapaths, Osteopaths, Faith Healers, Spiritualists, Herbalists, Christian Scientists, or MDs who use the brains they have, you never read about it in the big newspapers.

To teach the Rockefeller drug ideology, it is necessary to teach that Nature didn't know what she was doing when she made the human body. But statistics issued by the Children's Bureau of the Federal Security Agency show that since the all-out drive of the Drug Trust for drugging, vaccinating and serumizing the human system, the health of the American nation has sharply declined, especially among children. Children are now given "shots" for this and "shots" for that, when the only safeguard known to science is a pure bloodstream, which can be obtained only with clean air and wholesome food. Meaning by natural and inexpensive means. Just what the Drug Trust most objects to.

When the FDA, whose officials have to be acceptable to Rockefeller Center before they are appointed, has to put an independent operator out of business, it goes all out to execute those orders. But the orders do not come directly from Standard Oil or a drug house director. As Morris Bealle pointed out, the American Medical Association (AMA) is the front for the Drug Trust, and furnishes the quack doctors to testify that even when they know nothing of the product involved, it is their considered opinion that it has no therapeutic value.

PERSECUTION

Wrote Bealle:

"Financed by the taxpayers, these Drug Trust persecutions leave no stone unturned to destroy the victim. If he is a small operator, the resulting attorney's fees and court costs put him out of business. In one case, a Dr. Adolphus Hohensee of Scranton, Pa., who had stated that vitamins (he used natural ones) were vital to good health, was taken to court for 'misbranding' his product. The American Medical Association furnished ten medicos who reversed all known medical theories by testifying that 'vitamins are not necessary to the human body.' Confronted with government bulletins to the contrary, the medicos wiggled out of that one by declaring that these standard publications were outdated!"

In addition to the FDA, Bealle listed the following agencies having to do with "health"—i.e., with the health of the Drug Trust to the detriment of the citizens—as being dependent on Rockefeller: U.S. Public Health Service, U.S. Veterans Administration, Federal Trade Commission, Surgeon General of the Air Force, Army Surgeon General's Office, Navy Bureau of Medicine & Surgery, National Health Research Institute, National Research Council, National Academy of Sciences.

The National Academy of Sciences in Washington is considered the all-wise body which investigates everything under the sun, especially in the field of health, and gives to a palpitating public the last word in that science. To the important post at the head of this agency, the Drug Trust had one of their own appointed. He was none other than Alfred N. Richards, one of the directors and largest stockholders of Merck & Company, which was making huge profits from its drug traffic.

When Bealle revealed this fact, Richards resigned forthwith, and the Rockefellers appointed in his place the President of their own Rockefeller Institution, Detlev W. Bronk.

AMERICA'S MEDICO-DRUG CARTEL

The medico-drug cartel was summed up by J.W Hodge, M.D., of Niagara Falls, N.Y., in these words:

"The medical monopoly or medical trust, euphemistically called the American Medical Association, is not merely the meanest monopoly ever organized, but the most arrogant, dangerous and despotic organization which ever managed a free people in this or any other age. Any and all methods of healing the sick by means of safe, simple and natural remedies are sure to be assailed and denounced by the arrogant leaders of the AMA doctors' trust as fakes, frauds and humbugs.

Every practitioner of the healing art who does not ally himself with the medical trust is denounced as a 'dangerous quack' and impostor by the predatory trust doctors. Every sanitarian who attempts to restore the sick to a state of health by natural means without resort to the knife or poisonous drugs, disease imparting serums, deadly toxins or vaccines, is at once pounced upon by these medical tyrants and fanatics, bitterly denounced, vilified and persecuted to the fullest extent."

The Lincoln Chiropractic College in Indianapolis requires 4,496 hours, the Palmer Institute Chiropractic in Davenport a minimum of 4,000 60-minute classroom hours, the University of Natural Healing Arts in Denver five years of 1,000 hours each to qualify for a degree. The National College of Naprapathy in Chicago requires 4,326 classroom hours for graduation. Yet the medico-drug cartel spreads the propaganda that the practitioners of these three "heretic" sciences are poorly trained or not trained at all—the real reason being that they cure their patients without the use of drugs. In 1958, one of those "ill-trained" doctors, Nicholas P. Grimaldi, who had just graduated from the Lincoln Chiropractic College, took the basic science examination of the Connecticut State Board along with 63 medics and osteopaths. He made the highest mark (91.6) ever made by a doctor taking the Connecticut State Board examination.

COLONIZATION

Rockefeller's various "educational" activities had proved so profitable in the U S. that in 1927 the International Educational Board was launched, as Junior's own, personal charity, and endowed with $21,000,000 for a starter, to be lavished on foreign universities and politicos, with all the usual strings attached. This Board undertook to export the "new" Rockefeller image as a benefactor of mankind, as well as his business practices. Nobody informed the beneficiaries that every penny the Rockefellers seemed to be throwing out the window would come back, bearing substantial interest, through the front door.

Rockefeller had always had a particular interest in China, where Standard Oil was almost the sole supplier of kerosene and oil "for the lamps of China." So he put up money to establish the China Medical Board and to build the Peking Union Medical College, playing the role of the Great White Father who has come to dispense knowledge on his lowly children. The Rockefeller Foundation invested up to $45,000,000 into "westernizing" (read corrupting) Chinese medicine.

Medical colleges were instructed that if they wished to benefit from the Rockefeller largesse they had better convince 500 million Chinese to throw into the ashcan the safe and useful but inexpensive herbal remedies of their barefoot doctors, which had withstood the test of centuries, in favor of the expensive carcinogenic and teratogenic "miracle" drugs Made in USA, which had to be replaced constantly with new ones, when the fatal side-effects could no longer be concealed; and if they couldn't "demonstrate" through large-scale animal experiments the effectiveness of their ancient acupuncture, this could not be recognized as having any "scientific value." Its millenarian effectiveness proven on human beings was of no concern to the Western wizards.

But when the Communists came to power in China and it was no longer possible to trade, the Rockefellers suddenly lost interest in the health of the Chinese people and shifted their attention increasingly to Japan, India and Latin America.

THE IMAGE

"No candid study of his career can lead to other conclusion than that he is victim of perhaps the ugliest of all passions, that for money, money as an end. It is not a pleasant picture...this money-maniac secretly, patiently, eternally plotting how he may add to his wealth.... He has turned commerce to war, and honey-combed it with cruel and corrupt practices.... And he calls his great organization a *bene-faction*, and points to his church-going and charities as proof of his righteousness. This is supreme wrong-doing cloaked by religion. There is but one name for it—hypocrisy."

This was the description Ida Tarbell made of John D. Rockefeller in her "History of the Standard Oil Company," serialized in 1905 in the widely circulated McClure's Magazine. And that was several years before the "Ludlow Massacre," so JDR was as yet far from having reached the apex of his disrepute. But after World War II it would've been hard to read, in America or abroad, a single criticism of JDR, nor of Junior, who had followed in his father's footsteps, nor of Junior's four sons who all endeavored to emulate their illustrious forbears. Today's various encyclopedias extant in public libraries of the Western world have nothing but praise for the Family. How was this achieved?

Ironically, the two apparently most NEGATIVE events in the career of JDR brought about a huge POSITIVE change in his favor, to a degree that he himself could not foresee. To wit:

In the year when according to the current Encyclopaedia Britannica (long become a Rockefeller property and transferred from Oxford to Chicago), Rockefeller had "retired from active business," namely in 1911, he had been convicted by a U.S. court of illegal practices and ordered to dissolve the Standard Oil Trust, which comprised 40 corporations. This imposed dissolution was to provide his Empire with added might, to a degree that was unprecedented in the history of modem business. Until then, the Trust had existed for all to see—an exposed target. After that, it went underground, and thereby its power was cloaked in security, and could keep expanding unseen and therefore unopposed.

The second apparently negative experience was a certain 1914 event that persuaded JDR, until then utterly contemptuous of public opinion, to gloss over his own image.

"THE LUDLOW MASSACRE"

The United Mine Workers had asked for higher wages and better living conditions for the miners of the Colorado Fuel and Iron Company, one of the many Rockefeller-owned companies.

The miners—mostly immigrants from Europe's poorest countries—lived in shacks provided by the company at exorbitant rent. Their low wages ($1.68 a day) were paid in script redeemable only at company stores charging high prices. The churches they attended were the pastorates of company-hired ministers; their children were taught in company-controlled schools; the company libraries excluded books that the Bible-thumping Rockefellers deemed "subversive," such as "Darwin's Origin of the Species." The company maintained a force of detectives, mine guards, and spies whose job it was to keep the camp quarantined from the danger of unionization.

When the miners struck, JDR, Jr., then officially in command of the company, and his father's hatchet man, the Baptist *Reverend Frederick T. Gates*, who was a director of the Rockefeller Foundation, refused even to negotiate. They evicted the strikers from the company-owned shacks, hired a thousand strike-breakers from the Baldwin-Felts detective agency, and persuaded Governor Ammons to call out the *National Guard* to help break the strike.

Open warfare resulted. Guardsmen, miners, their women and children, who since their eviction were *camping in tents*, were ruthlessly killed, until the frightened Governor wired President Wilson for Federal Troops, who eventually crushed the strike, The New York Times, which then already could never be accused of being unfriendly to the Rockefeller interests, reported on April 21, 1914.

"A *14-hour battle* between striking coal miners and members of the Colorado National Guard in the Ludlow district today culminated in the killing of Louis Tikas, leader of the Greek strikers, and the destruction of the Ludlow tent colony by fire."

And the following day.

"*Forty-five dead (32 of them women and children)*, a score missing and more than a score wounded is the known result of the 14-hour battle which raged between state troops and coal miners in the Ludlow district, on the property of the Colorado Fuel and Iron Company, the Rockefeller holding. The Ludlow is a mass of charred debris, and buried beneath it is a story of horror unparalleled in the history of industrial warfare. In the holes that had been dug for their protection against rifle fire, the women and children died like trapped rats as the flames swept over them. One pit uncovered this afternoon disclosed the bodies of ten children and two women."

THOROUGH FACELIFT

The worldwide revulsion that followed was such that JDR decided to hire the most talented press agent in the country, Ivy Lee, who got the tough assignment of whitewashing the tycoon's bloodied image.

When Lee learned that the newly organized Rockefeller Foundation had $100 million lying around for promotional purposes without knowing what to do with it, he came with a plan to donate large sums—none less than a million—to well-known colleges, hospitals, churches and benevolent organizations. The plan was accepted. So were the millions. And they made headlines all over the world, for in the days of the gold standard and the five cent cigar there was a maxim in every newspaper office that a million dollars was always news.

That was the beginning of the cleverly worded medical reports on new "miracle" drugs and "just-around-the-corner breakthroughs" planted in the leading news offices and press associations that continue to this day, and the flighty public soon forgot, or forgave, the massacre of foreign immigrants for the dazzling display of generosity and philanthropy financed by the ballooning Rockefeller fortune and going out, with thunderous press fanfare, to various "worthy" institutions.

THE PURCHASE OF PUBLIC OPINION

In the following years, not only newsmen, but whole newspapers were bought, financed or founded with Rockefeller money. So Time Magazine, which Henry Luce started in 1923, had been taken over by J.P. Morgan when the magazine got into financial difficulties. When Morgan died and his financial empire crumbled, the House of Rockefeller wasted no time in taking over this lush editorial plum also, together with its sisters Fortune and Life, and built for them an expensive 14-story home of their own in Rockefeller Center—the Time & Life Building.

Rockefeller was also co-owner of Time's "rival" magazine, Newsweek, which had been established in the early days of the New Deal with money put up by Rockefeller, Vincent Astor, the Harrimann family and other members and allies of the House.

THE INTELLECTUALS—A BARGAIN

For all his innate cynicism, JDR must have been himself surprised to discover how easily the so-called intellectuals could be bought. Indeed, they turned out to be among his best investments.

By founding and lavishly endowing his Education Boards at home and abroad, Rockefeller won control not only of the governments and politicos but also of the intellectual and scientific community, starting with the Medical Power—the organization that forms those priests of the New Religion that are the modern medicine men. No Pulitzer or Nobel or any similar prize endowed with money and prestige has ever been awarded to a declared foe of the Rockefeller system.

Henry Luce, officially founder and editor of Time Magazine, but constantly dependent on House advertising, also distinguished himself in his adulation of his sponsors. JDR's son had been responsible for the Ludlow massacre, and an obedient partner in his father's most unsavory actions. Nonetheless, in 1956 Henry Luce put Junior on the cover of Time, and the feature story, soberly titled "The Good Man," included hyperboles like this:

"It is because John D. Rockefeller Junior's is a life of constructive social giving that he ranks as an authentic American hero, just as certainly as any general who ever won a victory for an American army or any statesman who triumphed in behalf of U.S. diplomacy."

Clearly, Time's editorial board wasn't given the choice to change its tune even after the passing of Junior and Henry Luce, since it remained just as dependent on House of Rockefeller advertising. Thus, when in 1979 one of Junior's sons, Nelson A. Rockefeller died—who had been one of the loudest hawks in the Vietnam and other American wars, and was personally responsible for the massacre of prisoners and hostages at Attica prison—Time said of him in it obituary, without laughing:

"He was driven by a mission to serve, improve and uplift his country."

Perhaps it was all this that Prof. Peter Singer had in mind when telling the judges in Italy that the Rockefeller Foundation was a humanitarian enterprise bent on doing good works. One of their best works seems to be sponsoring Prof. Peter Singer, the world's greatest animal friend and protector who claims that vivisection is indispensable for medical progress and for more than 20 years refuses to mention that legions of medical doctors are of the opposite view.

MILLIONS OF DOLLARS FREE PUBLICITY

Another interesting revelation in the article of Time was that many years ago already Singer "was pleasantly surprised when Britannica approached him to distill in about 30,000 words the discipline that is, at its heart, the systematic study of what we ought to do." So now we touch the subject of sponsorisation and patronage. They don't always mean immediate cash but, more important, long-term profits.

Many decades ago the Encyclopedia Britannica moved from Oxford to Chicago because Rockefeller had bought it to add much needed luster to the University of Chicago and its medical school, the first one he had founded. Peter Singer, "the world's greatest animal defender" who keeps a door permanently open to vivisection and the lucrative medical swindle, gets millions of dollars free publicity thanks to the worldwide engagement of the Rockefeller Foundation and the media-makers who are in no position to oppose it.

From the article in Time we also learned that Singer's mother had been a medical doctor in the old country, which could mean that little Peter started assimilating all the Rockefeller superstition on vivisection with his mother's milk.

Cited from the CIVIS Foundation Report number 15, Fall-Winter 1993

Reprinted with permission from CIVIS Foundation

The History of the Business with Disease

Matthias Rath, MD

The most powerful German economic corporate emporium in the first half of this century was the Interessengemeinschaft Farben or IG Farben, for short. Interessengemeinschaft stands for "Association of Common Interests" and was nothing other than a powerful cartel of BASF, Bayer, Hoechst, and other German chemical and pharmaceutical companies. IG Farben was the single largest donor to the election campaign of Adolf Hitler. One year before Hitler seized power, IG Farben donated 400,000 marks to Hitler and his Nazi party. Accordingly, after Hitler's seizure of power, IG Farben was the single largest profiteer of the German conquest of the world, the Second World War.

One hundred percent of all explosives and one hundred percent of all synthetic gasoline came from the factories of IG Farben. Whenever the German Wehrmacht conquered another country, IG Farben followed, systematically taking over the industries of those countries. Through this close *collaboration with Hitler's Wehrmacht*, IG Farben participated in the plunder of Austria, Czechoslovakia, Poland, Norway, Holland, Belgium, France and all other countries conquered by the Nazis.

The U.S. government investigation of the factors that led to the Second World War in 1946 came to the conclusion that *without IG Farben the Second World War would simply not have been possible.* We have to come to grips with the fact that it was not a psychopath, Adolf Hitler, or bad genes of the German people that brought about the Second World War. *Economic greed by companies like Bayer, BASF and Hoechst was the key factor in bringing about the Holocaust.*

No one who saw Steven Spielberg's film "Schindler's List" will forget the scenes in the concentration camp Auschwitz.

The Birth of I.G. Farben and the Support for Hitler (from the book Sword and Swastika by Telford Taylor)

After the First World War, all the major chemical concerns were merged in 1926 into a single gigantic trust—the I.G. Farbenindustrie A.G.—under the leadership of Carl Duisberg and Carl Bosch. Dyestuffs, pharmaceuticals, photographic supplies, explosives, and a myriad of other products poured forth in ever-growing volume and variety.

Soon after the election of July, 1932, in which the Nazis had doubled their vote, Heinrich Buetefisch [chief of the I.G. Farben—Leuna plant] and Heinrich Gattineau [a Farben official who was also an SA officer and personally known to both Rudolf Hess and Ernst Roehm] waited upon the Fuehrer-to-be to learn whether Farben could count on governmental support for its synthetic gasoline program in the event the Nazis should attain power. Hitler readily agreed that Farben should be given the necessary support to warrant expansion of the Leuna plant.

After the seizure of power, Farben lost no time in following up this auspicious introduction. Significantly, Farben's chosen channel was not the Heeresleitung but Hermann Goering's new Air Ministry. In a long letter to Goering's deputy Erhard Milch, Carl Krauch of Farben outlined a "four-year plan" for the expansion of synthetic fuel output. Milch thereupon called in Generalleutnant von Vollard Bockelberg, Chief of the Army Ordnance Office, and it was agreed that the Army and the Air Ministry together would sponsor the Krauch project. A few months later Farben received a formal Reich contract calling for the enlargement of Leuna so that production would reach three hundred thousand tons per year by 1937, with Farben's sales guaranteed for ten years—until June 30, 1944—on a cost-plus basis.

I.G. Farben and the Auschwitz Concentration Camp

Auschwitz was the largest mass extermination factory in human history, but the concentration camp was only the appendix.

The main project was IG Auschwitz, a 100% subsidiary of IG Farben, the largest industrial complex of the world for manufacturing synthetic gasoline and rubber for the conquest of Europe.

On April 14, 1941, in Ludwigshafen, Otto Armbrust, the IG Farben board member responsible for the Auschwitz project, stated to his IG Farben board colleagues, *"our new friendship with the SS is a blessing. We have determined all measures integrating the concentration camps to benefit our company."*

The pharmaceutical departments of the IG Farben cartel used the victims of the concentration camps in their own way: thousands of them died during human experiments such as the testing of new and unknown vaccines.

There was no retirement plan for the prisoners of IG Auschwitz. Those who were too weak or too sick to work were selected at the main gate of the IG Auschwitz factory and sent to the gas chambers. Even the chemical gas Zyklon-B used for the annihilation of millions of people was derived from the drawing boards and factories of IG Farben.

Medical Experiments in Auschwitz Conducted by I.G. Farben (from the book *I.G. Farben—from Anilin to Forced Labor* by Jorge Hunger and Paul Sander)

Scientific experiments were also done in other concentration camps. A decisive fact is that IG employee SS major Dr. med. Helmuth Vetter, stationed in several concentration camps, participated in these experiments by order of Bayer Leverkusen.

At the same time as Dr. Joseph Mengele, he experimented in Auschwitz with medications that were designated "B-1012, B-1034", "3382" or "Rutenol." The test preparations were not just applied to those prisoners who were ill, but also to healthy ones. These people were first infected on purpose through pills, powdered substances, injections or enemas. Many of the medications caused the victims to vomit or have bloody diarrhea. In most cases the prisoners died as a result of the experiments.

In the Auschwitz files correspondence was discovered between the camp commander and Bayer Leverkusen. It dealt with the sale of 150 female prisoners for experimental purposes: "With a view to the planned experiments with a new sleep-inducing drug we would appreciate it if you could place a number of prisoners at our disposal (…)"—"We confirm your response, but consider the price of 200 RM per woman to be too high. We propose to pay no more than 170 RM per woman. If this is acceptable to you, the women will be placed in our possession. We need some 150 women (…)"—"We confirm your approval of the agreement. Please prepare for us 150 women in the best health possible (…)"—"Received the order for 150 women. Despite their macerated condition they were considered satisfactory. We will keep you informed of the developments regarding the experiments (…)"—"The experiments were performed. All test persons died. We will contact you shortly about a new shipment (…)"

A former Auschwitz prisoner testified: "There was a large ward of tuberculars on block 20. The Bayer Company sent medications in unmarked and unnamed ampoules. The tuberculars were injected with this. These unfortunate people were never killed in the gas chambers. One only had to wait for them to die, which did not take long (…) 150 Jewish women that had been bought from the camp attendant by Bayer, (…) served for experiments with unknown hormonal preparations."

Parallel to the tests by Behringwerke and Bayer Leverkusen the chemical-pharmaceutical and serologic-bacteriological department at Hoechst started experimenting on Auschwitz prisoners with their new typhus fever preparation "3582". The first series of tests had results that were far from satisfactory. Of the 50 test persons 15 died; the typhus fever drug led to vomiting and exhaustion. Part of the concentration camp Auschwitz was quarantined, which led to an extension of the tests to the concentration camp in Buchenwald. In the journal of the "department for typhus fever and viral research of the concentration camp Buchenwald" we find on January 10th, 1943: "As suggested by the IG Farbenindustrie A.G. the following were tested as typhus fever medications: a) preparation 3582 <Akridin> of the chem. pharm. and sero-bact. Department Hoechst—Prof. Lautenschläger and Dr. Weber—(therapeutic test A), b) methylene blue, formerly tested on mice by Prof. Kiekuth, Elberfeld (therapeutic test M)."

The first and also the second series of therapeutic tests, held in Buchenwald between March 31st and April 11th 1943, had negative results due to insufficient contamination of the tested prisoners. Neither did the experiments in Auschwitz have evident successes.

The scientific value of all these experiments, whether ordered by the IG Farben or not, was in fact zero. The test persons were in bad physical condition, caused by forced labor, insufficient and wrong nutrition and diseases in the concentration camp. Add to this the generally bad sanitary circumstances in the laboratories. "The test results in the concentration camps, as the IG laboratory specialists should know, could not be compared to results made under normal circumstances."

The SS physician Dr. Hoven testified to this during the Nuremberg Trial: "It should be generally known, and especially in German scientific circles, that the SS did not have notable scientists at its disposal. It is clear that the experiments in the concentration camps with IG preparations only took place in the interests of the IG, which strived by all means to determine the effectiveness of these preparations. They let the SS deal with the—shall I say—dirty work in the concentration camps. It was not the IG's intention to bring any of this out in the open, but rather to put up a smoke screen around the experiments so that (…) they could keep any profits to themselves. Not the SS but the IG took the initiative for the concentration camp experiments."

The Nuremberg War Tribunal

The Nuremberg War Criminal Tribunal convicted 24 IG Farben board members and executives on the basis of mass murder, slavery and other crimes against humanity. Amazingly however, by 1951 all of them had already been released, continuing to consult with German corporations. The Nuremberg Tribunal dissolved the IG Farben into *Bayer, Hoechst, and BASF.*

Today each of the three daughters of the IG Farben is 20 times as big as the IG Farben mother was at its height in 1944, the last year of the Second World War.

More importantly, for almost three decades after the Second World War, *BASF, Bayer* and *Hoechst* (now *Aventis*) each filled its highest position, chairman of the board, with former members of the Nazi, NSDAP:

- *Carl Wurster,* chairman of the board of BASF until 1974 was, during the war, on the board of the company manufacturing Zyklon-B gas

- *Carl Winnacker,* chairman of the board of Hoechst until the late 70's, was a member of the Sturm Abteilung (SA) and was a member of the board of IG Farben

- *Curt Hansen,* chairman of the board of Bayer until the late 70's, was co-organizer of the conquest of Europe in the department of "acquisition of raw materials." Under this leadership the IG Farben daughters, BASF, Bayer, and Hoechst, continued to support politicians representing their interests.

During the 50's and 60's they invested in the political career of a young representative from a suburb of the BASF town of Ludwigshafen, his name: Helmut Kohl.

From 1957 to 1967 the young Helmut Kohl was a paid lobbyist of the "Verband Chemischer Industrie," the central lobby organization of the German pharmaceutical and chemical cartel. Thus, the German chemical and pharmaceutical industry built up one of its own as a political representative, leaving the German people with only the choice of final approval.

The result is well known: Helmut Kohl was chancellor of Germany for 16 years and the German pharmaceutical and chemical industry became the world's leading exporter of chemical products, with subsidiaries in over 150 countries, more than IG Farben ever had. Several billion people will now die prematurely, if the pharmaceutical industry gets its way. Germany is the only country in the entire world in which a former paid lobbyist for the chemical and pharmaceutical cartel was head of the government. In summary, the support of German politics for the global expansion plans of the German pharmaceutical and chemical companies has a 100-year-old tradition.

It is with this background that we understand the support of Bonn for the unethical plans of the Codex Commission. (Remark made by the Dr. Rath Health Foundation)

The U.S. lead prosecutor in the Nuremberg War Criminal Tribunal against the IG Farben anticipated this development when he said, "these IG Farben criminals, not the lunatic Nazi fanatics, are the main war criminals. If the guilt of these criminals is not brought to daylight and if they are not punished, they will represent a much greater threat to the future peace of the world than Hitler if he were still alive."

The Disgraced Managers of I.G. Farben

Fritz ter Meer (1884-1967)

- Member of the IG FARBEN executive committee 1926-1945, member of the working committee and the technical committee, director of section II

- 1943 plenipotentiary for Italy of the Reich Minister for armaments and war production, military economist chief industrialist responsible for Auschwitz.

- 1948 found guilty of "plundering" and "enslavement" and condemned to seven years detention. Released 1952.

- 1955 board member of Bayer

- 1956-1964 chairman of the board of Bayer chairman of the board of Th. Goldschmidt AG, deputy chairman of the board of Commerzbank bank association AG, board member of the Waggonfabrik Uerdingen, the Duesseldorfer waggonfabrik AG, the bank association West Germany AG and the United Industrial enterprises AG (VIAG)

Otto Ambros (1901-)

- Member of the IG FARBEN executive committee 1938-1945, member of the chemical committee and chairman of commission K (agents), special advisors of Krauchs F+E department for the four-year plan, director of the special committee C (chemical agents), the main committee for powders and explosives in the office for arms, military industrial leader

- Responsible for choice of location, planning, building and running of IG Auschwitz as operations manager. Managing director of the Buna-Works and synthetic fuel production

- 1945 knight's cross Distinguished Service Cross

- 1948 found guilty of "enslavement" condemned to eight years detention.

- Released 1952.

- Starting from 1954 chairman, deputy chairmen and member of the boards of: Chemie Grünenthal, Pintsch Bamag AG, Knoll AG, Feldmühle Papier-und Zellstoffwerke, Telefunken GmbH, Grünzweig & Hartmann, Internationale Galalithgesellschaft, Berliner Handelsgesellschaft, Süddeutsche Kalkstickstoffwerke, Vereinigte Industrieunternehmungen (VIAG) with its daughter enterprises Scholven-Chemie and Phenol-Chemie as an advisor to F. K. Flickund of the US Industrialist J.P. Grace is entangled in the early eighties in the "Flick scandal"

Hermann Schmitz (1881-1960)

- Member of the IG FARBEN executive committee 1926-1935, chairman of the board 1935-1945 and "chief of finances" to the IG

- Military industrial leader, member of the Nazi party (NSDAP)

- 1941 war Distinguished Service Cross 1st. Class

- 1948 found guilty of "plundering" condemned to four years prison.

- Released 1950.

- 1952 board member of the German bank Berlin West

- 1956 honorary chairman of the board of Rheini steel plants.

Fritz Gajewski (1888-1962)

- Member of the IG FARBEN executive committee 1931-1945, leader of section III (coordination with Dynamite Nobel)

- At Nuremberg, found "not guiltily" for all charges

- 1949 managing director, 1952 chairman of the board of Dynamite Nobel AG

- 1953 Distinguished Service Cross of the Federal Republic of Germany

- 1957 retirement, honorary chairman of the board of Dynamite Nobel AG, chairman of the board of Genschow & Co. and the Chemie-Verwaltungs AG, board member of Huels AG and the Gelsenkirchener mines

Heinrich Buetefisch (1894-1969)

- Member of the IG FARBEN executive committee 1934-1945, deputy director of section I, director of gasoline synthesis for IG Auschwitz

- 1932 (together with Gattineau) had the conversation with Hitler, that defined the petrol pact, 1936 co-worker of Krauch on the four year plan as a production representative for Öl in the Arms Ministry

- SS Obersturmbannführer, military industrial leader, awarded the "friend of the Reich leader SS" cross.

- 1948 found guilty of "enslavement" condemned to six years detention.

- Released 1951.

- 1952 supervisory board member of Ruhr-Chemie and Kohle-Öl-Chemie among others.

- 1964 Distinguished Service Cross of the Federal Republic of Germany. The award was taken back after 16 days due to the violent protests

Friedrich Jaehne (1879-1965)

- Member of the IG FARBEN executive committee 1934-1945, chief engineer of the IG, deputy director of the BG central Rhine/Maingau

- 1943 military industrial leader, Distinguished Service Cross 1st. Class 1948 found guilty of "plundering" condemned to 18 months detention

- 1955 supervisory board member of the "new" Farbwerke Hoechst. In the same year elevated to supervisory board chairman elect—Karl Winnacker said "in the meantime the liquidation conclusion law had been issued and freed us from all discriminating regulations. So we could add Friedrich Jaehne, chief engineer of the old IG, to the supervisory board. He presided over this committee until 1963. None of us would have thought in 1945 that we would come to such a co-operation."

- Supervisory board chairman of the Alfreds Messer GmbH (late Messer Griesheim), supervisory board member with Linde

- 1959 Dr. Ing. E.h. of TH Munich, 1962 Bayer service medal, honorary senator of TH Munich, Distinguished Service Cross of the Federal Republic of Germany

Carl Krauch (1887-1968)

- Member of the IG FARBEN executive committee 1926-1940, chairman of the board 1940-1945, director of the coordination center W, director of the Reich office for economics, plenipotentiary for special questions on chemical production, military industrial leader.

- 1943 knight's cross for distinguished service.

- 1948 found guilty of "enslavement" and condemned to six years prison.

- Released 1950.

- 1955 board member of Huels GmbH.

- In the Frankfurt 1956 Auschwitz court case is quoted as saying: "they were usually anti-social elements so called political prisoners" (describing the prisoners of Auschwitz-Monowitz)

Carl Wurster (1900-1974)

- Member of the IG FARBEN executive committee 1938-1945, director of BG upperRhine, board member of DEGESCH

- Military industrial leader and Reich calculation chamber of economics

- 1945 knight's cross Distinguished Service Cross

- At Nuremberg, found "not guiltily" of all charges

- 1952 chairman of the board of the "new" BASF, chairman of the board for Duisburger Kupferhuette and Robert Bosch AG, board member of Augusts Viktoria, the Buna-Werke Huels GmbH, the Süddeutschen Bank, Deutschen Bank, Vereinigten Glanzstoff, BBC, Allianz, Degussa, 1965 retirement as chairman of the board of BASF

- 1952 honorary professor of the University of Heidelberg, Dr. rer. RK h.c. the University of Tübingen, 1953 Dr. Ing. E.h. of the TH Munich, 1955 Distinguished Service Cross of the Federal Republic of Germany, Bayer service medal, 1960 Dr. rer. pole h.c. the University of Mannheim, honorary senator of the Universities of Mainz, Karlsruhe and Tübingen, honorary citizen of the University of Stuttgart, honour citizen of the city of Ludwigshafen, 1967 Schiller prize of the city of Mannheim, president of the federation of the chemical industry, vice-president of the Max-Planck company, the company of German chemists.

From "Arbeit macht frei" to "Codex Alimentarius"

Just fifteen years after they were convicted in the Nuremberg War Crimes Tribunal, Bayer, BASF and Hoechst were again the architects of the next major human rights offences. In 1962, they established the Codex Alimentarius Commission. (*Remark made by the Dr. Rath Health Foundation*)

This dark period of German history is inextricably bound to one man, Fritz ter Meer:

- He was a member of the Managing Board of IG Farben from its inception to its dissolution. As the Wartime Manager, he was responsible for IG Auschwitz.

- In the Nuremberg Tribunal, ter Meer stated: "Forced labor did not inflict any remarkable injury, pain, or suffering on the detainees, particularly since the alternative for these workers would have been death."

- In 1948, ter Meer was sentenced by the Nuremberg Tribunal to seven years in prison for plundering and slavery.

- In 1952, his sentence was commuted, due to the influence of powerful friends.

- From 1956-1964, he was reinstated as a member of the Managing Board of Bayer AG.

- In 1962, ter Meer was one of the architects of the "Codex Alimentarius"—Commission and one of the main designers of the schemes that would profit from human suffering. (*Remark made by the Dr. Rath Health Foundation*)

The deceptive title "Codex Alimentarius" is no accident. It was devised by the same firms and indeed the same individuals, who gave the Auschwitz concentration camp inmates the deceptive slogan "Arbeit mach frei" ("Work makes you free"). (*Remark made by the Dr. Rath Health Foundation*)

Reprinted with permission from the Dr. Rath Health Foundation, USA

References

Chapter 1: Cancer at a Glance

1. Rath, Mathias. *Cellular Health Series: Cancer.* Santa Clara: MR Publishing, 2002.

2. Pollick, Michael. *What is Cancer?* [Updated 2006; cited 15 May 2006]. Available from http://www.wisegeek.com/what-is-cancer.htm

3. Ibid

4. Adachi, Ken. *Cancer.* [Updated 26 February 2002; cited 20 May 2006]. Available from http://educate-yourself.org/cancer/

Chapter 2: The business of Healthcare

1. Adachi, Ken. *Forbidden Cures.* [Updated 31 December 2005; cited 20 May 2006]. Available from http://educate-yourself.org/fc/ (**This chapter reprinted with permission from Ken Adachi**)

2. W. Hoffman, *David: Report on a Rockefeller.* New York: Lyle Stuart, Inc., 1971. page 24

3. Adachi, Ken. *Forbidden Cures.* [Updated 31 December 2005; cited 20 May 2006]. Available from http://educate-yourself.org/fc/

4. Ibid

5. Ibid

6. Ibid

7. Ibid

8. Ibid

9. Ibid

Chapter 3: A New Perspective on Health and Disease

1. Erasmus, Udo. *Fats that Heal, Fats that Kill.* Burnaby: Alive Publishing, 1993.

2. Ibid

3. Appleton, Nancy. *Rethinking Pasteur's Germ Theory: How to Maintain Your Optimal Health.* Berkeley: Frog Ltd. Publishing, 2002.

4. Ibid

5. Bland, Jeffrey, Linda Costarella and Buck Levin. *Clinical Nutrition: A Functional Approach.* Gig Harbor: The Institute for Functional Medicine, 1999.

6. Erasmus, Udo. *Fats that Heal, Fats that Kill.* Burnaby: Alive Publishing, 1993.

Chapter 4: The Standard American Diet (SAD)

1. Erasmus, Udo. *Fats that Heal, Fats that Kill.* Burnaby: Alive Publishing, 1993.

2. Ibid

3. Weston Price Foundation. *Real Milk is Not Pasteurized.* [Cited 20 May 2006]. Available from http://www.realmilk.com/what.html

4. Ibid

5. Trudeau, Kevin. *Natural Cures "they" Don't Want You to Know About.* Elk Grove: Alliance Publishing Group, Inc., 2004.

Chapter 5: Environmental Hazards

1. Steinman, David. *Diet for a Poisoned Planet: How to Choose Safe Foods for You and Your Family.* New York: Harmony Books, a Division of Crown Publishers, 1990.

2. Ibid

3. Steinman, David, and Samual Epstein. *The Safe Shopper's Bible: A Consumer's Guide to Nontoxic Household Products.* New York: Wiley Publishing, Inc., 1995.

4. Rubin, Jordan. *The Maker's Diet*. Lake Mary: Siloam Publishing, 2004.

5. Trudeau, Kevin. *More Natural "Cures" Revealed*. Elk Grove: Alliance Publishing Group, Inc., 2006.

6. Ibid

Chapter 6: Modern Society Pays a Heavy Price

1. Murray, Michael, and J. Pizzorno. *The Encyclopedia of Natural Medicine*. Rocklin: Prima Publishing, 1998.

2. Rubin, Jordan. *The Maker's Diet*. Lake Mary: Siloam Publishing, 2004.

3. Schweitzer, Albert, in his preface to A. Berglas, *Cancer: Cause and Cure*, as quoted in James South "Laetrile—The Answer to Cancer." [Cited 12 May 2006]. Available from http://www.antiaging-systems.com/extract/laetrile.htm

4. Stefanson, Vilhjalmur. *Cancer: Disease of Civilization*. New York: Hill and Wang Publishing, 1960.

5. Dewailly, E., et al., "High Organochlorine Body Burden in Woman with Estrogen Receptor-Positive Breast Cancer," *Journal of the National Cancer Institute* 86 [February 2, 1994]: 232-234

Chapter 7: The Essentials of Health and Healing

1. Goldberg, Paul. *Hygienic heights: Public Health, Source oriented Gastroenterology, Clinical Nutrition and Health Related Issues of Women and Men from a Biological—Hygienic Perspective*. Marietta: Published by Paul Goldberg, 2002.

2. Lipski, Elizabeth. *Digestive Wellness*. Los Angeles: Keats Publishing, 2000.

3. Ibid

4. Appleton, Nancy. *Lick the Sugar Habit*. Santa Monica: Avery Publishing, 1996.

5. Erasmus, Udo. *Fats that Heal, Fats that Kill*. Burnaby: Alive Publishing, 1993.

6. Ibid

7. Ibid

8. Bland, Jeffrey, Linda Costarella and Buck Levin. *Clinical Nutrition: A Functional Approach.* Gig Harbor: The Institute for Functional Medicine, 1999.

9. Roberts, H.J. *Aspartame (NutraSweet): Is it safe?* Philadelphia: The Charles Press Publishers, 1992.

10. "Saccharin Stays on Carcinogen List." *The Lancet,* (1997;350:1300), Morbidity and Mortality Weekly Report, (1996;45:207-209).

11. *Fact vs. Fiction: The Truth about Splenda.* [Cited 18 May 2006]. Available from http://www.truthaboutsplenda.com/factvsfiction/index.html

12. Blaylock, Russell. *Excitotoxins: The Taste that Kills.* Santa Fe: Health Press, 1997.

13. Erasmus, Udo. *Fats that Heal, Fats that Kill.* Burnaby: Alive Publishing, 1993.

Chapter 8: Everything in the Universe is Energy

1. Wikipedia. Albert Einstein. [Updated 25 May 2006; Cited 26 May 2006]. Available from http://en.wikipedia.org/wiki/Albert_Einstein

2. *The Secret.* Produced by Rhonda Byrne and directed by Drew Heriot. 89 min. Prime Time Productions, 2006. DVD.

Chapter 9: The Universal Law of Attraction

1. Trudeau, Kevin. *Natural Cures "they" Don't Want You to Know About.* Elk Grove: Alliance Publishing Group, Inc., 2004.

2. Emoto, Masaru. *The Hidden Messages in Water.* Tokyo: Sunmark Publishing, Inc. 2001

3. Ibid

4. *The Secret.* Produced by Rhonda Byrne and directed by Drew Heriot. 89 min. Prime Time Productions, 2006. DVD.

Chapter 10: The Secret to Attracting Vibrant Health

1. Dyer, Wayne. *The Power of Intention.* Carlsbad: Hayhouse, 2004.

978-0-595-40169-7
0-595-40169-4

Printed in the United States
59475LVS00003B/112-114